ENOUGH
ABOUT THE
BABY

ENOUGH ABOUT THE BABY

A BRUTALLY HONEST GUIDE TO SURVIVING THE FIRST YEAR OF MOTHERHOOD

BECKY VIEIRA

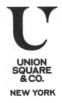

UNION
SQUARE
& CO.

NEW YORK

UNION SQUARE & CO.

NEW YORK

UNION SQUARE & CO. and the distinctive Union Square & Co. logo
are trademarks of Sterling Publishing Co., Inc.

Union Square & Co., LLC, is a subsidiary of Sterling Publishing Co., Inc.

The information in this book is intended for informational or educational purposes
only. This book is not intended or implied to be a substitute for professional medical
advice, diagnosis or treatment. All content, including text, graphics, images, and
information contained herein is for general information purposes only and is
offered with no guarantees. The author and publisher disclaim all liability in
connection with the use of this book and the material it contains. The author and
editor have made every effort to reproduce the substance of the conversations relied
on in this book but some have been edited and condensed for clarity and space.
Some names and identifying details have been changed at the individuals' request.

ISBN 978-1-4549-4799-8 (paperback)
ISBN 978-1-4549-4800-1 (e-book)

For information about custom editions, special sales, and premium purchases,
please contact specialsales@unionsquareandco.com.

Printed in Canada

2 4 6 8 10 9 7 5 3 1

unionsquareandco.com

Interior design by Rich Hazelton

For Archie.
I love you more,
I love you most,
It's a tie!

Contents

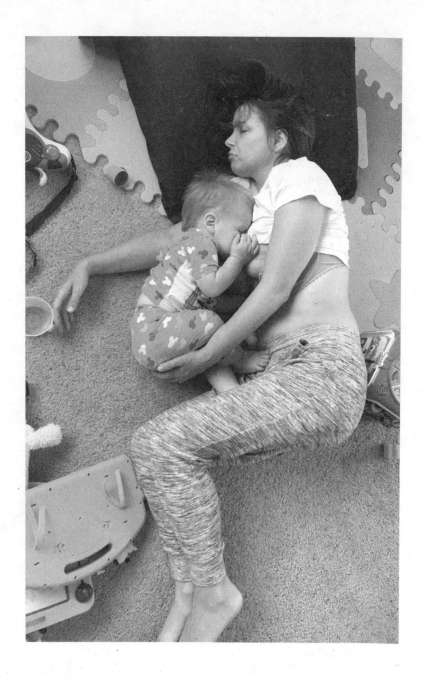

INTRODUCTION

A friend of mine gave birth about a month before my due date. She was understandably busy, and it wasn't until a few weeks after her daughter was born that we finally connected. I expected to hear a typical recap of her time since the birth of her daughter: that she was tired, recovering from childbirth, but also deliriously happy and madly in love. Isn't that what all new moms say?

She said nothing of the sort.

"It's been awful," she began. "Don't get me wrong—I love my baby. But it's nothing like I expected."

She went on to tell me that she was exhausted in a way she never thought possible and actually didn't trust herself to drive a car. Her husband had returned to work, and she struggled to find time just to eat. She'd taken to shoving lone pieces of turkey lunch meat into her mouth as sustenance. She was in pure survival mode and she sounded scared and unsure of herself—like she knew she was teetering on the edge of a cliff but didn't know how to step back and find safer ground.

I was shocked. I'd never heard anyone speak of motherhood like this before. Of course, I knew it was hard. But this?

She sounded like an overexaggerating drama queen. I felt sorry for her that she was experiencing such a struggle, but I just knew it wouldn't be like that for me. After all, she was the first person I'd ever heard describe motherhood in that way. Maybe her hormones were surging after giving birth and clouding her opinion, right?

Wrong. After I had my son, Archie—now six years old—I felt just about the same as my miserable friend, but wondered why we were the only two mothers who appeared to feel this way. Or, if not, why hadn't anyone else told me the full truth?

I don't think anyone was trying to deliberately deprive me of this information; a lot of new mothers forget the early days once they move into the next stage of motherhood. Sharing the harsh realities of those first months seems less important once they end. Women have long joked that their brain blocks out the hard parts of labor and delivery; otherwise they'd never want to have a child again—and there may be some truth to this. Plenty of research suggests that the various biological changes happening during pregnancy appear to have an impact on brain function, especially memory.

In short: Our bodies might actually be trying to focus our brains on the good parts so that we will have another baby and continue the human race. But it's more complex than that, of course.

The universal nature of motherhood also seems to work against us. Instead of women banding together in solidarity about how difficult and challenging motherhood is, there is an attitude of "Everyone has done it, so it can't be that bad." The moms who came before us didn't discuss the dirty details and therefore many can't understand why this generation wants to. They didn't talk about the pain of that first postpartum poop or how you feel existential panic about the thought of never being able to leave the house again without an overflowing diaper bag. Their mothers never told them, so they aren't telling us. They stayed silent and got through it and they're leaving us to do the same.

These women might want us to follow suit and keep silent because it's generational and they just don't believe that women should discuss feeling depressed or the pain of cracked nipples. Or perhaps there is a sense of jealousy that keeps them quiet: They weren't able to openly share their struggles, so why should you get to? Ultimately, motherhood is seen by these previous generations as your "job," no matter how hard or messy it may get. Just as they once did, we are expected to keep our heads down, keep our mouths closed, and get to work.

I'm not here to do a sociological study on why this silence is the norm, but rather to say that healthy conversation about all aspects of motherhood is vital to our well-being. Women have been conditioned to keep the challenging aspects of motherhood quiet, and in order to change that reality, we need to first become aware of it.

Some women will flat-out scold others for talking about the difficulties, telling them they'll scare people away from becoming moms. Others will be more subtle, cutting your story off midway and changing the subject, or recalling their own "wonderful experience," intended to shame you into silence if yours was anything less than magical. It's a gut punch when you first realize that some women, especially other moms, don't want you to be honest.

I remember one day at the park when another mom asked me how I was, and I began to answer her honestly. "I'm scared that I'm messing up," I said. "And yesterday, he had a diaper blowout that went all the way up the back of his onesie that I didn't even notice for twenty minutes." Her eyes darted away from mine, and she said nothing. I quickly picked up on the fact that this conversation was intended to be a cursory interaction. She didn't really want to know how I was; she just asked to be polite.

And that wasn't the last time. It happened with other moms on playdates, at Mommy & Me classes, with my closest friends and neighbors, and even while talking with older, extended family during holiday dinners. "Well," they'd say in a condescending tone, "*we've* all been there, and *we've* all managed to survive." In other words, "Shut up, kid."

Staying quiet about our true experiences is not helping anyone. It merely makes the journey much more difficult—and lonelier—than it needs to be.

In addition to generational and societal expectations, today's moms also have social media to contend with. And it's not making things any easier for us.

For example, when I'm having a bad day as a mom, I often find myself getting short on patience with my son, and I sometimes cry or go to bed early. My house probably looks like it hosted a weeklong retreat for a group of gorillas, and I'll serve cereal for dinner before I declare that bedtime will be one hour earlier than usual. Then, after I've managed to get Archie to bed, I turn to social media for reassurance that I'm not alone. There is a strong chance I'll come upon the page of a "mom influencer" whose day looks nothing like mine. She'll post a picture of her and her immaculately dressed (and matching) five children sitting in an entirely white and spotless kitchen with a caption that says something like, "You know I will always keep it real and be honest with you. Today was one of my hardest days as a mama to these five kids. That's why I'm going to share my secret with you. When times get tough and I want to cry, I love to reset my mindset by going into the kitchen with all my kids and baking **INSERT BRAND NAME HERE** cookies together. #Ad"

It's not a total lie, that *is* a picture of her baking with her kids. But what we don't see is everything else that is happening beyond the camera's frame. There could be piles of laundry, a stained couch, and a sixth child in the midst of a meltdown.

Social media allows users to choose what other people see, and it's up to us to wade through the filters and find "real" moms online. Moms who don't bake cookies in a clean kitchen on hard days, moms who share how they yelled at their kids and cried and felt like a failure.

I wanted to become one of *those* moms, the ones who are honest about motherhood. I started sharing my story through articles and soon turned to social media, where I was one of the imperfect moms talking not only about the good parts, but also about the days I yelled and cried. I found an immediate connection with other moms who had the same experiences.

Seeing firsthand how moms find solace in hearing about the hard times—because it tells them they aren't alone and their feelings are common—is what led me to write this book. It's everything I wish I had known about the first year of motherhood. I've spoken with hundreds of other mothers, plus doctors, nurses, and experts in breastfeeding, baby sleep, family therapy, and even car seat installation, and it's all here to help guide you on the path I wish I had walked after my son was born. It's everything new moms need to talk about but usually don't.

Motherhood is harder than you think, in every respect. And better, too.

Beyond embracing the honesty that we not only crave but also need, we must step forward and advocate for ourselves as women and mothers. If we don't, no one else will. And we'll go about our lives sacrificing our own health and happiness for that of our children, partners, and everyone else. It's entirely possible to be a great mother and still have your needs met. Unfortunately, society is not yet ready to offer that to us, which is why we must demand it—starting with our partners and those around us.

You'll notice mothers are often called superheroes, as if we're a wonder to behold (we are). I actually believe society started calling us that because it was easier for everyone around us to sit back and let us carry the load while making it seem like they're complimenting us—rather than actually stepping up to help us and taking anything off our plates.

It's okay to be selfish. It's okay for this journey to also be about you. In fact, you and your baby will actually thrive if you let yourself do that.

The baby is going to be just fine. Now let's focus on you.

Introduction

A Disclaimer about Terminology: *I know that all families are unique, and are made in different yet equally beautiful ways. Not all parents are married or live under the same roof. Some families have two moms, others two dads. There are single parents, adoptive and foster parents, stepparents, and parental figures. And moms have different co-parents: wives, husbands, girlfriends, boyfriends, partners, and more. I am not able to duplicate this colorful list with each reference and will refer to this person as "partner." When telling my own story, I will use the term "husband" because that is what I have.*

A Disclaimer about Medical Advice: *I am an advocate for moms, someone with her ear to the ground and helping to drive the motherhood revolution forward. I am not a doctor. I am also not a nurse, a psychologist, a psychiatrist, a therapist, a counselor, a midwife, a doula, a lactation consultant, a sleep consultant, or a certified car seat technician. To find reliable and detailed medical information, you can refer to* Resources and Further Reading *(page 310). It's important to always speak with a physician about your health concerns and before making any medical decisions.*

Introduction

A Disclaimer about the Birthing Process and Care Providers: *While the location where pregnant people give birth isn't limited to a hospital's delivery room, nor are care providers strictly doctors and nurses, the majority deliver at hospitals under the care of a medical team, as was my experience. As such, I have chosen in the first two chapters to focus specifically on delivery and recovery in hospital settings.*

CHAPTER 1
Your Hospital Stay

The baby has exited your body. Now what?

"What does he look like? Does he have hair?" I asked my husband as I scanned the room in hopes of seeing my newborn baby. Considering that my body was numb from the waist down and I could only lift my head a few inches up from the bed (or was it an operating table?) where I lay as the doctor stitched me back together, there wasn't much chance that I'd be able to spot a tiny baby from my current vantage point.

"He has hair," my husband answered, his gaze laser-focused on the corner of the room where I could only guess he was looking at our child. "And it's dark," he added.

Great, I thought. *A baby with dark hair.* But when would I see him? Why wasn't anyone showing him to me? It's not like I expected my doctor to hold him above her head like baby Simba in *The Lion King* as soon as he emerged from my body, but I assumed someone would have given me a glimpse of him by now. After all, I'd just spent 39.4 weeks creating him inside my uterus. Didn't that automatically qualify me for VIP viewing status? Apparently not.

I assumed that I wasn't intentionally being deprived of seeing my baby, but I also didn't know what was happening at the time.

I later learned that this was common and that the medical team was assessing my baby's Apgar score, which is an evaluation done at birth. It checks a baby's color, heart rate, reflexes, muscle tone, and breathing rate.

And so it went on for a while after that. My husband preoccupied by the baby in the corner. My doctor periodically checking in on me as she pieced my body back together. And me, alone with my thoughts. I didn't cry. Wasn't I supposed to cry? Did that say something about the type of mother I am? Nothing was going as I expected. Granted, those expectations were based on things I'd seen on TV and in movies.

I didn't speak up because I felt like an uninvited observer. Doctors and nurses looked to be busy doing official, important tasks. It didn't seem as if I should interrupt them, so I stayed silent. I wish I could go back and tell myself to use my voice and ask for what I wanted because I missed so much of that monumental life moment. And I didn't have to stay silent. I just wasn't aware of what typically happens in the moments right after giving birth.

Little did I know that would be the first in a long list of things I wish someone had told me about motherhood. Things that could have made my entire journey completely different.

And better.

As most moms will tell you, giving birth and meeting your new baby will be more powerful than you ever imagined. You've spent around forty weeks preparing as best you can to make everything perfect. You've researched car seats, taken classes, attended dozens of doctors' appointments, written a birth plan, and done everything you could think of to prepare for welcoming your child into the world—including taking excellent care of yourself during pregnancy. After all, you were the vessel that protected your child as they grew from that tiny speck you squinted to identify during your first ultrasound.

As a woman over the age of thirty-five, my pregnancy was deemed "geriatric," and it unfolded under the very watchful eye of several medical professionals. I was at my doctor's office about three times a week in the final trimester.

Once I gave birth it ended abruptly. I knew it was no longer about me. It didn't have to be, not entirely. But it should have been, just a bit.

Once your body is no longer a protective growth container, do you immediately forgo your own health and well-being? No, absolutely not. You shouldn't neglect what you need while you're in the hospital, and you certainly don't have to. But you might have to get a little "selfish," meaning you will need to advocate for yourself. Because as soon as that beautiful baby arrives, you will fall into a distant second place in terms of importance. And you might feel like you're being selfish by making even your most basic needs known, but I promise you that's not true. Your baby deserves a happy and healthy mother. And you deserve to enjoy your new role. Unfortunately, there is no guarantee that all your needs will be

---

EXPERT TIP

Birth trauma is real and comes in many forms. You do experience some loss of control over your body during childbirth, and having knowledge of what is going on will help you to feel more comfortable. Ask your doctor to walk you through the process of labor and delivery and what will be happening at each step. Try to visualize what it will look like. If you have specific wants in the delivery room, it doesn't hurt to ask your doctor. Generally, we try to accommodate anything that isn't going to have a negative impact on your health. The ultimate decision can be hospital-specific for what is allowed, such as music or a photographer, and I highly recommend that you also ask about any wants during your labor and delivery tour.

—Christine Sterling, MD, ob-gyn

---

met unless you step forward and take control, which is something you'll need to do at the moment when you're most vulnerable.

Back in that operating room, where my son had just been delivered, my teeth had begun to chatter and I noticed that my legs, which were still numb from the epidural, were shaking. It was surreal. There was activity all around me, but no one seemed to actually *see* me. Was this what an out-of-body experience felt like? It was as if I were watching the scene unfold from afar, not as a key participant. I felt bile begin to curdle in the back of my throat. "I'm going to be sick," I said, though not loudly enough for anyone to hear me. I tried again. "I AM GOING TO BE SICK!" I said, this time with what felt like a very dramatic emphasis. I felt guilty that, in the midst of all the important things everyone was doing, someone was now going to have to stop to help me.

A nurse appeared at my side with what looked like a medical-grade barf bag, which she held under my mouth. I began to throw up and heard her and my doctor discuss which medication I would need for what appeared to be a reaction to the anesthesia. At this point I just wanted to sleep.

Less than five minutes later, another nurse stepped over and placed my son on my chest. "Here he is," she said. I'd spent months imagining what he would look like and how it would feel to hold him, and now the moment had finally arrived. Yet I was so nauseated that I just stared at him, waiting for some emotion to take over. My husband was gazing down at us with tears in his eyes. But all I felt was the need to continue vomiting.

I wrapped my arm around my son, surprised at how tiny he was, especially next to my breast that was newly engorged to twice the size of his head. I felt like I should do something unforgettable, so I looked at him and said, "Hi. We're your parents. We're probably going to embarrass you at some point, but know we always love you." The room erupted in laughter, and I felt pleased with myself. The reaction made me feel like I'd done something right.

He looked so fragile and helpless, but he somehow started scooting his body across my chest like an inchworm. "He's ready to breastfeed!" someone said with a strange sense of excitement, but I just laughed. There was no way this was going to happen now, especially with my body still trying to expel any remaining bile in my stomach. I was wrong.

One nurse held my baby to my breast while another kept that barf bag squarely under my mouth. His tiny mouth that looked so helpless only a moment ago had encircled my nipple with what felt like a death grip. And did he have saliva in his mouth or was that acid? Because it felt like acid.

"Help," I whispered.

"One minute, mama. We just have to get this little guy fed first, then we'll take care of you," someone (barf bag nurse, maybe?) said. "But you're doing so great!"

I was happy that my son was getting the care and attention he needed. But it felt like a bucket of cold water being thrown in my face as someone quickly kicked me out of the medical care cocoon in which I'd been safely ensconced for nine-plus months. I realized that he would not just be *a* priority; he'd be *the* priority. I wanted him to get everything he needed, all the care and attention. I suppose I just expected that I'd get some, too.

If I had to pinpoint the exact moment when I knew I was on my own, it was when they took me to my hospital room after my delivery, where my mom greeted me. "Since you're

---

EXPERT TIP

We call the first hour after childbirth the "golden hour" and that is when you want to try to get a newborn baby to latch. Lately, I've seen that stretched to within the first two hours if the mother and baby practice skin-to-skin contact as soon as possible. However, when it comes to mothers who have a C-section, there is the understanding that this can be delayed, and, in most cases, babies who are delivered via C-section rarely eat during the golden hour. I look at the golden hour as being primarily about uninterrupted skin-to-skin time with early breastfeeding initiation being a secondary benefit. Skin-to-skin is recommended for both breast- and formula-feeding moms because of the amazing benefits. So, yes, a baby can wait to nurse, especially if the mother is feeling sick. Mothers always have a say in the first feed; we always have a right to advocate for ourselves.

—Leah Castro, certified lactation consultant

---

okay, do you mind if I go and see my new grandson?" she asked. "They said I can hold him now!" Even in my hazy state I could hear the excitement in her voice. I mumbled something affirmative and off she went.

While in my room, I tried to sleep while enduring what felt like an endless loop of breastfeeding and various doctors, nurses, and hospital staff coming in to check on the baby. As postpartum hospital stays go, mine was fairly uneventful, in that there were no complications or emergencies, just a lot of unknowns. So after hearing from hundreds of my fellow mothers, I've compiled a comprehensive list of the things you should probably know before going to the hospital.

1. Uterine massages (sometimes referred to as "fundal" massages) may be part of your recovery.

Don't get excited by my use of the word *massage*. This one will be the antithesis of everything you've come to know that word to mean. I promise that, contrary to how it may feel, this is not conducted as a means of torture. It's done to prevent bleeding and promote contracting of the uterus after childbirth. It will feel like someone has climbed to the top of the Empire State Building and dropped a bowling ball directly onto your midsection. Several times a day. You may not experience a fundal massage, but if you do, don't feel like you have to suffer. According to Dr. Christine Sterling, "You can ask for a break from uterine massages unless your care team is seeing excess bleeding."

2. Both your baby and you will be wearing diapers.

You will be wearing an industrial-strength adult "diaper" that is usually made up of a maxi pad the size of a pool float and a pair of mesh "granny" panties. You need all this because of postpartum bleeding and the shedding of lochia. It won't be light spotting; the inside of said "diaper" will look like a crime scene. So will the toilet and shower each time you use either one. And the lochia, which is made up of bits of your insides that are slowly shedding away from within your body, will smell like bits of your insides that are slowly shedding away.

3. A lot of people will be coming into your room at various times for different reasons.

A group that feels twice the size of the population of New York City will be parading in and out of your room. Taking blood, testing the baby's hearing, talking to you about birth certificates and social security cards and 7,614 other things. They have no shame; they won't wait for you to cover up or stop crying. And if you are asleep, don't worry . . . they'll abruptly turn on the lights and wake you up. This is their job. They've seen it all and are professionals, so what may feel like a shocking intrusion to you is all in a day's work for them.

I assumed that I had to let every person who sashayed through that door come in and do exactly what they came to do, right at that moment. And in some cases, yes, you do—and for various reasons. Perhaps the task needs to be done immediately, or maybe the person doesn't have time to come back later. But there are times when it's nothing urgent. You won't know unless you or your partner asks.

4. Even though your visitors mean well, you still might need a safe word.

Yes, your family and friends will want to meet your new bundle of joy and overload you with flowers. And more flowers. But remember: This time in the hospital is intended for you to recuperate. If that means cutting your aunt's visit short, so be it. Also, some visitors can't take a hint when you are ready for them to leave. Talk with your partner in advance of your hospital stay and come up with a code word that means "Kindly get them out of here." And enlist your nurses, too. They don't want guests setting up shop in your tiny hospital room any more than you do.

5. Your baby will be less calm on night two.

After the haze of delivery fades, your baby will come alive. Loudly and frequently. My husband and I actually asked our nurse if they accidentally switched babies on us, and we were only half joking. Some people call this "hell night" or "second night syndrome," and it is said to be the result of your baby realizing that they are now in a new environment and no longer safely ensconced in your uterus. It is normal, but it can be alarming if you're not expecting it. Be prepared to give extra comfort and hold your baby a little longer when this happens, and you'll probably lose a little more sleep.

Real Mom Story

My husband kept asking how to help. There wasn't much I needed at the moment, but I was about to go to the bathroom and that is a whole process in itself. I asked him to get my "bathroom gear" ready for me: fresh water in my peri bottle, a new pad, and a clean pair of mesh panties. He gathered everything and set it up next to the toilet for me, then called me in when it was ready.

I sat down to tend to my battered baby chute with my peri bottle. As I started to pee, I squeezed the water and screamed. It was quite possibly the hottest water ever known to man. Truly, he must have run off when I wasn't looking and found a hot spring because it felt like a steaming geyser was now spraying my vagina.

My husband ran into the bathroom and asked me what was wrong. "It's BOILING hot," I yelled. "Do you not remember what just happened to this area of my body?" He looked at me, confused. "Yes, that's why I thought you'd want hot water. It's more sterile."

At that point there was nothing I could do except laugh. I also made sure not to assume my husband knew exactly what I needed, and to be very specific when I asked for help. And not just with him, with everyone.

—Ashley B.

6. There may be more help available than you realize.

I wasn't even aware that there was a nursery available for my baby: I thought he had to stay in my room the entire time because no one told me otherwise. Instead of sleeping, I spent a lot of the first night staring at him to make sure he was breathing. If I'd known, I would have asked for him to go to the nursery for at least a few hours so I could let someone else be responsible for monitoring his breathing. Also, you don't have to send your baby to the nursery if you don't want to. It's your baby and you get to choose where they sleep.

It's worth noting that some hospitals have recently started to eliminate nurseries altogether in favor of babies rooming with their parents, so this may not even be an option to consider when you give birth. But you can and should ask. And even if there's no nursery, ask your nurse if there is any time when they can take your baby to give you a quick break, whether to sleep, shower, or just be left alone.

Many nurses I spoke with said they are always happy to do what they can to help, when there is time, but that also means you need to be on good behavior. "It's not that hard to be a good patient," one nurse told me. "Treat us with the same respect you'd want, understand that we're busy and trying our best, and don't act as if we're servants—we are highly trained and educated medical professionals. I always give all my patients the same level of care because that's my job. But I'm more likely to give 'extras' to the ones who are appreciative and respectful."

7. It may be uncomfortable to urinate at first.

It will feel like a flow of hot lava is pouring from your vagina. Use the squirt or "peri bottle" while you pee to help soothe things down there. And also, before and after you use the restroom. Then take it home with you and never let it out of your sight. And, speaking of time spent in the bathroom, the aftermath of your first shower may look like a massacre just took place. It's helpful to take your first postpartum shower at the hospital, because they have industrial-strength cleaning products there.

8. Your first days of breastfeeding will unfold with an audience.

Remember when we talked about all those people coming in and out of your room? Well, I assumed that if I was breastfeeding when any of them arrived, they'd quickly leave and return later. Wrong. Breastfeeding will not deter anyone from entering your room, even some of those friends and relatives whom you'd rather not be familiar with the shape and shade of your areolas. There's nothing quite like a stranger making direct eye

Real Mom Story

Just as I drifted off to sleep after feeding my baby on our first night in the hospital, the lights in the room came on and a nurse entered. "Bath time," she announced. I was so disoriented that I thought she meant a bath for me. I quickly realized she meant my daughter, who was still sleeping. I looked at the clock and was surprised to see it was 1 a.m.

My husband and I looked at one another, and he shrugged, as if to say, "I guess we're doing this." I was unable to get out of bed, so the nurse had him assist with the bath. But first, he had to wake up our sleeping newborn baby, which caused her to scream. Loudly. And the screaming continued throughout the entire bath.

The nurse left us with a clean but hysterical baby and told us to get some sleep. I guess she didn't realize that was exactly what we'd been trying to do!

If I knew that I could have, I would have asked the nurse to come back and let us sleep. In fact, eighteen months later, when our second daughter was born, the hospital staff informed us that they no longer bathed newborns, just cleaned them up after delivery. Imagine that.

—Candice A.

contact with you as you breastfeed for the first time ever in your life. By the time I left the hospital I think there was only one gift shop employee who hadn't seen my boobs. But it's okay. No one really looks and, eventually, you don't even care if they do. It's actually quite liberating.

9. Those candid postpartum photos aren't really candid at all.

We've all seen those photos of women cradling their newborn baby where everything looks effortless. And perfect. She is wearing a cute hospital gown with flawless hair and makeup as she gazes adoringly at her child. Do not be alarmed if you don't look like this after delivery. These women didn't either. They flat-ironed their hair, contoured their face, and probably had a professional photographer with them.

I had a scheduled C-section, which allowed me to shower, do my hair, and put on a little makeup before I arrived at the hospital. But by the time I was back in my room with my baby, I looked like I'd brushed my hair with an eggbeater, and there was no sign of makeup to be found. I was so tired and sore that I no longer cared.

And those cute gowns and pajamas? A lot of women sweat and have hot flashes after birth, due to hormones. Plus, you'll be bleeding and wearing diapers. If I was going to sweat and bleed on anything, it was going to be the hospital's gown. Not mine.

10. You can never be too prepared.

There is a difference between what you *need* while you are in the hospital and what you'll *want* to make your stay more enjoyable. And both are equally important. To help you prepare, see The Ultimate Hospital Packing List (page 275).

CHAPTER 2

Your Hospital Discharge

It's not a hotel.
There's no late checkout and you need to leave.

In just a few hours I'd be set free from the hospital. I'd become accustomed to knowing that a team of professionals was within earshot should anything go wrong. The fact that this was ending—and I was now expected to know how to be a mom—wasn't sitting well with me. But for now, I was safe and protected . . . in a hospital bathroom.

I braced myself as best I could and stepped into the shower. I kept the bathroom door open in case I fell or needed help, but, luckily, this was a hospital, and the shower came complete with a safety bar that I held onto. Besides, I can't imagine anyone would want to see what was happening in there. I didn't even want to see it.

No sooner had I stepped under the stream of water when things started falling out of me. Out of my vagina, specifically. Blood, clumps of tissue I couldn't identify, and more blood. It smelled strongly of copper pennies in that way blood usually does. I closed my eyes and tried to forget about it and enjoy the shower. Aside from the pain in my incision, this was the first time since my son was born that something actually felt good—not counting when the pain meds kicked in, that is. In that moment the shower was better than any spa treatment, and I felt somewhat renewed.

I turned the water off and looked around. My insides were everywhere. It looked like I'd barely survived an attempted murder.

I called my mom in and insisted that we try to clean up because I couldn't let anyone see. She made a good effort, but it looked like an industrial cleaning would be in order. She helped me put on my "going home" outfit: a "mom diaper" and a loose-fitting maternity dress. I squeezed my ham-hock feet, which were triple their normal size due to all that fluid retention, into a pair of my husband's slippers, which seemed to be the only footwear that would fit me.

It was time for my hospital discharge. I was exhausted, in pain, and scared. I asked my husband if we could cash in the college savings account we'd started and instead hire a nurse to live with us for the rest of our lives. Or until the money ran out.

I didn't want to leave the hospital because then I'd be on my own. When my doctor came by to clear me for discharge, I reminded her that at some point she had mentioned that I might need to stay a fourth night, though I couldn't remember why. It didn't matter. I was desperate. If she had said it was for a colonoscopy, I would have gladly rolled over and spread my butt cheeks right then and there.

"I considered having you stay an extra day because you were retaining so much fluid," she explained. "But it's leveled off now. You can go home! Be with family and enjoy your new baby."

She said it like my going home was a good thing.

Dr. Sterling later told me that doctors look for specific things before a new mom will be discharged. "The bleeding should be under control, and she can eat and drink. For C-section moms, we want them to be passing gas. And all vital signs should be normal."

I met all the discharge criteria and she signed off on my exit. This was the time my anxiety escalated from "Oh crap, I have to go home and be responsible for my newborn baby!" to "OH CRAP, I HAVE TO GO HOME AND BE RESPONSIBLE FOR MY NEWBORN BABY!"

I was expecting my husband to be on the same page as me and agree that leaving the hospital that day was bonkers. He should have been telling my doctor this or calling our insurance company to get approval for me to stay another day. Instead, he yawned before agreeing with my doctor that going home would be a good thing. Was he insane?

I've come to realize a lot since that day, specifically that my husband's wants or needs shouldn't have come before my own. Granted, this isn't a contest of "which parent is more exhausted," but mothers are the ones who give birth, so don't ignore their requests, no matter how ridiculous they may seem in the moment.

EXPERT TIP

Some hospitals make parents bring a car seat into the room to prove that you have one and make sure you know how to harness your baby in the seat. Others want to see it in the car itself. Even if you aren't planning to ever transport your child in a car, most hospitals will still require this to determine if your baby can tolerate sitting in a semi-reclined position. If your baby's oxygen levels drop during the test, that means they shouldn't be using ANYTHING that keeps them at a similar angle, like the bouncy seat, swing, and some strollers, until your pediatrician clears them for that (usually weeks or months later). Ask the labor and delivery unit of the hospital about its car seat policy before you give birth.

Families leaving on a bus or train with a newborn aren't required by state law to use a car seat (there could always be the rare exception) because there are no seat belts or latch anchors to secure the car seat.

Depending on your state, taxis might be classified as commercial vehicles; therefore, the use of a car seat may not be required. Please always use one. When you call for your taxi, let the dispatcher know that you will be using a car seat. Uber, Lyft, or anything similar are treated the same as a personal vehicle under state law and require the use of an appropriate car seat. Make a note of this when you request the car.

—Jessica Choi, child passenger safety instructor

After the yawning incident, I dressed my son in the lamb onesie and sweater that I'd chosen for his coming-home outfit. I loved it a week ago but seeing it on him now, I realized he looked like a little old gnome dressed up for Easter. I didn't have a second outfit option, so I had little choice other than to hand my gnome-lamb-baby to my mom while my husband packed up my things. My dad was back at our house, assembling the bassinet that had, of course, arrived *after* I'd given birth.

Our nurse arrived with my discharge instructions and even more paperwork, brochures, and forms to add to the stack that had been growing steadily each day we'd been there.

My husband had brought our car seat up to the room earlier and, in the presence of one of our nurses, I gingerly placed my newborn inside and secured the straps. I think I would have been calmer if I was dismantling a live bomb.

My son began screaming and turned bright red. His face contorted with each wail, and I was reminded once again that newborns rarely look like the babies you see in movies and on TV. Sure, there are always outliers, the ones who actually *do* look as if they're headed to a Gerber baby photo shoot straight out of the uterus (one of my closest friends birthed three of these). But mine didn't. He was slightly jaundiced, had black sideburns, a nose that seemed a few sizes too big for his face, and a little scratch on his cheek from his razor-sharp newborn fingernails that made him look like he'd been involved in a baby gang fight. But he was *my* little gang member.

Although my son actually had a fairly round head, some babies don't at first. They can be born with misshapen heads. But don't worry: That's completely normal. According to Dr. Sterling, "a newborn's skull is not yet fused because it needs to fit through the pelvis during a vaginal delivery." The head will mold to the size of the pelvis so it can squeeze through, and that can often result in a baby having a conehead shape upon delivery. It's not permanent; Dr. Sterling says this will only last about forty-eight to seventy-two hours. And, no, you aren't imagining it if your baby doesn't look exactly as you expected. "Newborn babies are often very pink, their skin can peel, and they might have acne or cradle cap," she explains. "Their face may have been squished when they went through the pelvis, and they could even be hairy those first days or weeks. Whatever the case, the baby you give birth to will look completely different in four weeks."

It's okay if you think your newborn looks odd or not like what you expected. A lot of moms feel that way, I promise you. Many of us look back and joke about it. They eventually gain more weight and will morph into one of those plump and delicious babies that you had envisioned.

After our car seat was approved, we removed our howling child from its grip and my mom held him as I tried to settle into a wheelchair for my exit scene. I groaned and winced, as I had with every movement for the past three days, because my midsection, which felt like it had been sliced open, had recently been sliced open. My mom gently rubbed my back. My husband yawned. I seethed inside.

My baby was placed in my arms and again I wondered how anyone thought it was a good idea that I be in charge of this tiny human. My husband left with the car seat and would be bringing our car to the front of the hospital to pick us up, and with that we were off. I was wheeled out by a hospital employee, baby in my arms and my mom walking with us. It felt surreal, like I was hyperaware of a disaster about to happen and no one else could see what was coming. How could they act so casual?

The baby went back into the car seat, the car seat went into the car, and I somehow contorted my still-healing body into the back seat next to him. My mom left in her car, and we followed behind with a planned stop at a pharmacy to pick up my pain medications. "We didn't take any pictures of us leaving the hospital," I said, on the verge of tears. "Me, him . . . in the wheelchair. Leaving." My husband reassured me that we had plenty of photo opportunities ahead of us, but I was crushed that we had missed that one. So much so that I started crying. In the moment it felt like one of my life's greatest failures.

We pulled into the pharmacy parking lot and my husband went inside. I just stared at my son, hoping he'd give me a clue as to what I was supposed to do with him. Here we were, two people who were literally connected to one another just days before, and I felt as if we were strangers. It started to feel awkward, so I grabbed my phone and started taking pictures of him so I wouldn't have to think. I was grateful when my husband returned and I was no longer alone with my own child. A child I now had seventy-plus more photos of than I had six minutes before because, again, I didn't know how to coexist with my own baby.

We returned home and, to my delight and surprise, my parents were waiting in the driveway with a bouquet of "It's a boy" balloons tied to the porch railing. My dad was filming our arrival and captured everything from our car pulling up to us walking through the front door. I had never realized it, but I desperately wanted that greeting and those balloons. Luckily, my mom is big on celebrations. Those balloons may have been a small gesture, but they felt like the world to me. That, and my dad's camera skills, helped ease some of the sting of not capturing our hospital exit.

Looking back now, it's clear that a lot of my disappointment and sadness was likely due to hormones. Everything seemed to be a bigger challenge than it normally would have, my tears came quickly, and I wasn't as open to reason or logic as I'd been a week before. Those hormone changes hit me, and they hit hard. Every woman is different, but for those who feel seemingly uncontrollable feelings, as I did, go easy on yourself. You're not being dramatic or overreacting. Given everything your body and

Real Mom Story

On my discharge day, I felt like the staff were trying to push me out the door faster than I was ready. I was trying to get together with the lactation consultant, which was taking longer than expected, and we'd been given a specific cutoff time for our stay that was now creeping up on us. The whole process felt rushed, and I started to panic. I wasn't ready to leave, and the pressure was making me feel even more uncertain about what to do when we got home.

When we started packing up to go, my baby was crying and hungry. I must have looked panicked because my wife told me to sit down and just feed the baby. She would take care of the nurses, she said. I was so grateful to her at that moment. I always tell friends who are expecting to ask for what you need in the hospital. If you feel like the nurses or doctors aren't hearing you, ask again. If your baby is crying or you need a few more minutes to regroup, it's okay. Leaving the hospital is overwhelming enough on its own. Don't let the perception of pressure from the staff make it harder on you.

—Cait G.

brain are going through, it's no wonder a balloon could make you cry. As Dr. Sterling told me, "Nothing compares to the hormonal shift that occurs after birth, not the beginning of pregnancy, not puberty, not menopause—it is profound. Hormones impact our mood, emotions, and behavior. We feel this abrupt decrease in hormones and for many it does not feel good."

Leaving the hospital with my new baby actually reminded me of going off to college. I went from being a high schooler living at home with a curfew to suddenly being expected to manage my life as a grown adult without the guidance of the parents who had been with me for the past eighteen years. It's jarring, and a bit scary. There are things I wish I knew beforehand that will hopefully ease this process for you, and I've listed them here.

1. You will be given a lot of papers that matter.

There will be a lot of paperwork leaving the hospital with you— pamphlets, leaflets, and brochures. Some of it is very important; other forms and brochures are nice to have. I mistakenly chose to keep all of mine in one massive, disorganized stack, which forced me to shuffle through it more often than I'd expected. Here is what you will want to prioritize:

- Information on how to obtain your baby's birth certificate and social security card. Many hospitals will help you complete one or both of these before your discharge. In my experience, we had to request the birth certificate through our county's website, but some hospitals will give you the form.

- Information on postpartum depression, such as signs to look for and resources. I thought I didn't need this, until I did. I scrambled to find it in the middle of the night and was unsuccessful. If I had to do it all over again, I would have had this in an easily accessible place.

- Medical information, such as warning signs to watch for in the health and recovery of both you and your baby, when to call a doctor or 911, and general tips.

- Information on feeding and assistance for either breast-feeding or formula feeding (it doesn't matter how you feed your baby, as long as it is what YOU think is best for the two of you), plus information on how to obtain a breast pump through your insurance company or rent one from the hospital.

- Resources, including for advice hotlines, support groups, lactation consultants, therapists, and any person or organization that might help you in your postpartum journey.

- Appointment reminders for your baby's pediatrician visits. There will be a few in the first weeks after birth.

- Various tip sheets, including safe sleep, car seat safety, and notes on any medication you or your baby will be taking.

- Less essential, but helpful for many, are feeding and pooping/peeing charts. This is an easy way to track your baby's activity to know that they are eating enough and also having everything coming out the other end as frequently as it should.

2. Ask questions until you feel like you're annoying people. And then ask some more.

Many new moms are anxious about leaving the hospital because they will no longer have immediate access to doctors, nurses, and various baby experts. So why not ask those people as many questions as you can while you are only a call button away? There are no stupid questions, and if anyone makes you feel that way, just ignore them and ask again. You are preparing to be wholly responsible for a newborn baby and most likely not thinking much about your own recovery. That is massive. Ask away! Write down questions as you think of them, both before and during your stay. Whatever is easiest for you, whether it be on paper, in your phone, or even as a voice memo. You can even come to the hospital with a list of outstanding questions from your pregnancy. If you are too tired, sick, or busy, ask your partner, a family member, or a nurse to help. (See page 283 for a list of questions you might want to consider asking before your discharge.)

3. You might care more than you think about what your baby wears home.

Yes, as in what the baby will wear as they depart the hospital. For some it's almost ceremonial, the first "real" clothes they'll wear; others like it for photo purposes. I suppose it was a bit of both for me, and I have my son's outfit saved with some other memories like his hospital ID bracelet. It's a good idea to have a backup in case something happens to the clothes or if you change your mind. It doesn't hurt to store them safely (perhaps in a bag inside your hospital bag), and to make sure anyone who might help you dress your baby knows what you want them to wear.

4. Be the squeaky wheel.

I am not good at asking for things, but many of my friends are. That's how they came home from the hospital with extra diapers, wipes, peri bottles, mesh granny panties, onesies, baby blankets, and hats. Ask what extras you can take home. The worst they can say is "nothing," though I've heard tales of new moms leaving with enough diapers to last two weeks. And in terms of diaper costs, that's worth a lot.

5. Your only responsibility is to yourself and your baby.

There can be a lot going on at this time. Pass off as much as you can to others so that all you need to do is go home. Straight home, preferably. Try to envision what you might need when leaving and in the twenty-four hours that follow, and ask someone (a partner, a family member, or a friend) to get what they can ahead of your discharge. I was in a lot of pain when I left the hospital and wish I had skipped the stop at the pharmacy. It's an errand my husband could have managed alone before we went home. Do you need formula or wipes? Is someone going to be in your yard blowing leaves when you get home, keeping you from sleeping? Cancel or reschedule things that may interfere with the first days home, like a gardener or housekeeper. Start a list before your baby is born and amend it as needed during your hospital stay. Also, think about what is waiting for you when you finally do arrive home. I had a scheduled C-section, so I knew exactly when I was leaving my house to give birth. Not everyone has that luxury. Maybe your baby was born early and you didn't have everything ready, or your labor progressed so quickly that you left for the hospital with a carton of milk on the kitchen counter. Whatever it might be, you certainly don't need to deal with it when you get home.

6. You might go home while your baby stays in the hospital.

No one wants to think about this, but it's a reality for some parents. Whether you know in advance of your delivery that your baby will need to stay in the NICU (neonatal intensive care unit) for medical reasons, or it transpires while you are there, it's a gut-wrenching scenario. It's important to realize that your baby will receive the best care possible from staff who are highly trained and will also love and advocate for your baby as their own. You can—and should—proactively ask for updates, whether you are

EXPERT TIP

Having a baby in the NICU is incredibly stressful and very emotional. I had two babies in the NICU, and I've never been more scared in my life. Seeing your sweet baby hooked up to tubes for breathing and feeding is frightening. I recommend talking to your health care provider to get an idea of what you can anticipate. How long do they think your baby will be in the NICU? What is the progression you can expect? What milestones are they looking for as you are ready for discharge? I found a timeline detailing when you can take them home very valuable.

Don't be afraid to speak up. Doctors and clinicians want to hear your questions. I love when parents come to appointments with lists. We can review each one, and it makes for a more efficient and successful visit.

It is helpful to talk to NICU parents who have been there longer than you, as their baby is likely progressing and working toward discharge. You also need to enlist the help that will be offered back home. Ask someone to pick up groceries, do a load of laundry (or take your wash to the laundromat), and throw some meals in the freezer. These are not things you will be eager to do with sleep deprivation and this emotional roller coaster.

Also, know that most babies leave the NICU within a few days and grow and develop as usual. My own babies' admissions were devastating, but they are now healthy and happy boys.

—Dina Kulik, MD, FRCPC, Pediatrics

in the NICU or calling to check in. NICUs provide support and many have resources that may include free cafeteria meals and a place to comfortably stay overnight and shower. But that doesn't mean you should live there. Most of all, it's important to remind yourself that you are not to blame for this. Write it on Post-it notes and stick them everywhere: This Is Not Your Fault.

7. Someone will talk to you about postpartum depression and mental health, and you need to listen.

You will meet and speak with a lot of people during your stay and as you prepare to leave. But you will also be exhausted and out of sorts during many of those conversations, so it's hard to keep track of all the information that is coming your way. One of those people will be there to speak with you about postpartum depression and maternal mental health. LISTEN TO THIS PERSON. My mental health felt no different than usual during my hospital stay; if anything, I was on a bit of a high—figuratively and literally— because I was on pain medication after having my C-section. I'll be honest: What I was hearing sounded like an improbable reality. Yes, I was weepy and emotional, but this was many levels beyond that. I didn't pay that much attention and accepted the paperwork I was given and added it to my stack. Please, pay attention. Listen, ask questions, and read whatever you are given. Be aware of the signs to look for, what to do if you start to feel depressed, or even different than you usually do, which

I will go into in greater detail in Chapter 9: Your Emotional Health (page 181). Know how and where to get help. In the best-case scenario, you never have to use the information.

8. You might not be able to wear your own clothes when you go home.

Each postpartum body is unique and special—and hard to predict. I had originally packed some loose maternity lounge pants to wear home, but the thought of having anything with a waistband in the vicinity of my incision made me cringe. Plus, my milk had come in and my breasts were big. Very big. Too big for me to be comfortable in the shirt I had planned to wear. I was ready to leave in a hospital gown until my mom went to my house and picked up one of my maternity dresses.

9. A shot list for photos is not a dumb idea.

I was already writing for a baby website when I gave birth, so my editor and I talked about what type of photos I might take during my hospital stay that would be good for upcoming articles. But I didn't think beyond the time inside the hospital itself and missed out on photos I desperately wished we had (such as that hospital exit shot). Think of everything that might be happening and what you'd like to capture and make a list. My husband and I made a video for our son outside the hospital before we walked in, telling him we love him and can't wait to meet him. It's short

Real Mom Story

We live in a big city and don't own a car, so we used Uber to get home from the hospital. We didn't prepare; we just requested a car once we were in the hospital lobby and assumed all would be fine. It wasn't. Our Uber driver had no idea where the car seat latches and anchors were and he was beyond irritated that he had to wait while we fumbled around with a car that was foreign to us. He eventually told us to call someone else and left. Many infant car seats can be installed without the base and just using the car's seat belt, but I didn't know that at the time.

My advice to anyone in this situation is to be clear that you will have a car seat when calling your Uber. Before you give birth, practice using the seat belt to install the car seat so that you don't feel overly pressured by the audience of the Uber driver. Borrow a friend's car or take some Uber practice runs to install the seat.

Also, don't close the door until the baby seat is installed. The Uber can't drive away until the doors are closed, and this gives you the power to decide when you're ready to go.

And be sure to tell the driver that you need time and thank them for their patience up front. Kindness always goes far.

—Darcie T.

and simple, but my son loves watching it now that he's older. Maybe you want to ensure that absolutely no photos are taken of you in those mesh granny panties. Whatever it may be, list your do's and don'ts for photos. Most important, get in the pictures yourself. It's easy to dismiss these opportunities, especially when you don't feel comfortable with your body or how you look in that moment, but these are times you will never get back. Your baby will never again be a few days old.

10. There's a strong possibility that the drive home will cause anxiety.

The simple act of placing your tiny, helpless, and vulnerable newborn baby in a car is nerve-racking in itself, but when that car actually starts moving on a road—with other cars—it's downright terrifying. And, unless you live close enough to walk home, you will check off the "baby's first car ride" milestone on this day. My husband drives, as our son and I love to tell him, "like a ding-dong." He can make me nervous even in the best of situations, so I asked him ahead of time not to drive on the freeway and to resist every impulse he felt to drive anywhere other than the slow lane. Plan your ride home in advance and choose streets with less traffic or maybe even a route that avoids the highway. A lot of women actually drive the route in advance to make sure they feel comfortable with it. The more say you have in the trip, the better you will feel.

CHAPTER 3

Your First Few Days at Home

Congratulations! You're now solely responsible
for a tiny, helpless human.

O n my last morning in the hospital, my doctor noticed a small rash on my midsection. By the time I arrived home later that same day, it had spread rapidly and was covering about 60 percent of my body. I'd developed a systemic allergic reaction that would proceed to work its way through my entire body. I'm talking between my fingers and toes and inside my ears. It caused my body to swell and itch uncontrollably.

It was never determined what exactly I was allergic to, but I was prescribed prednisone, a corticosteroid used to treat many things, including inflammation caused by allergies. It was also perfectly safe to continue breastfeeding while on the dosage I was prescribed. After about a week, the rash cleared up and I've never had any reactions since.

I wouldn't worry too much about this happening because it's neither common nor specific to my C-section. I'm just telling you about it because the pain of this rash led me to experience one of the most cringe-worthy moments in my life, which happened on the day I came home from the hospital with my baby.

We'd been home only an hour or two and I felt miserable. The rash was brutal, and I was ready to rip my skin off. I think it's only because I was too tired to physically scratch my skin into oblivion that I didn't. On top of that, my engorged breasts, which were full of all that breast milk that had now officially come in, felt like a geyser about to blow at any moment.

I remembered when a friend, who had a baby about four years earlier, had mentioned having that similar "something is about to pop" feeling when her milk came in. She said one day she was so desperate that she sat topless in the sun and it worked better than any heating pad at releasing some of the pressure in her milk ducts. I was desperate, so I decided to give it a try. I told my husband and parents in no uncertain terms not to go into the backyard and placed a patio chair out of sight from any windows, stripped down to my pad-lined granny panties from the hospital, and slowly lowered myself into the chair. The relief was instantaneous: Somehow that sunshine sent healing rays upon my angry breasts and I felt a moment of peace.

And then I heard, "Excuse me? Ma'am?"

I quickly jumped up (except it wasn't quick at all because I could still barely move, thanks to my incision) and covered my chest with my arms. It was the gardener, who was there for his weekly yard maintenance. I was so out of it that I'd completely lost track of the day and time. I apologized profusely, put my head down, and waddled back inside while a stream of pee slid down my leg. It wasn't one of my finer moments, though it is one of the more unforgettable.

Some people gently ease into being at home with a newborn, but not me. I got things started by giving a poor stranger a disturbing and unrequested postpartum peep show *with* a side of golden shower. And that was the beginning of my life at home with a newborn.

It's important to talk about the first few days at home, separate from anything else, because that initial time can be brutal. These days are not like the first weeks or months when changing diapers becomes second nature and you know how to hold your baby to best comfort them. No, right now you have no idea what you are doing, and you're probably scared silly. It's the hardest and most intense on-the-job training that you'll ever have. It's like someone said, "Since you read these baby books, we'll go ahead and give you a tiny newborn who is entirely helpless. Have fun!" Not only do you need to get through these first few days of survival as best you can, but your hormones will be doing backflips while your body heals. It's intense.

"This is a tough time," agrees Dr. Kulik. "We are all nervous about bringing home a newborn. In fact, when we brought our first baby home, I was in my final year of pediatrics residency, and even I was scared. It is a steep learning curve that every new parent must face and adapt to. You can never be prepared for the exhaustion and emotional roller coaster of new parenthood."

Real Mom Story

We were mostly prepared to have our son come home. What we didn't prepare for was the actual act of getting home. We live in a third-floor walk-up apartment in a big city. With no elevator. We took a cab to the hospital, and my boyfriend had rented a car to take us home. He double-parked in front of our apartment and helped me and our baby inside, then had to run off to park the car. I just stood there thinking, *What am I supposed to do now?* When he returned, we started up the stairs, me leading the charge and my boyfriend behind me carrying our son in his car seat. I was making slow progress up the stairs. Everything hurt, and it felt like an inferno inside the stairwell. As soon as we finally passed the first floor, our son started screaming. I started crying because I assumed that I was a horrible mother for letting him cry. My boyfriend tried to soothe him while I tried to walk faster, but that only resulted in me peeing my pants. I had a massive pad on, but I guess it wasn't meant to hold blood and a full bladder. At that point I just gave up and, down on my hands and knees, crawled up the dirty and disgusting stairs. I really wish we had put some thought into how we would actually get into our home. We could have enlisted friends to help.

—Sabita K.

Coming home from the hospital, as in actually walking into my home with a new baby in tow, wasn't what I expected. I assumed it would feel massive, like I was stepping into the next chapter of my life. But it was quiet and uneventful, not unlike when I'd walked through the same door less than a week before with groceries. It was hard to reconcile how our home could feel the same, yet my mind and body felt entirely foreign to me.

I hadn't wanted to leave the hospital, but after three days in a small hospital room, I had started to feel almost caged in. Not only physically, but emotionally as well. It was like I'd lost all bodily autonomy after giving birth. True, I wasn't being forced to have anything done against my will—and I have the utmost appreciation and respect for the doctors and nurses who treated me, and I know everything was done for my health and benefit— but after having things done for and to me, I was feeling almost claustrophobic and needed space around me.

Aside from my backyard rendezvous with the gardener, I spent the next few days existing between breastfeeding sessions. That time was when I would try to eat, use the bathroom, or sleep. Relaxing was difficult because I had a constant fear that something would happen to my baby that I couldn't put aside.

One thing that really took me by surprise was how much time would be spent breastfeeding. Not only the act itself, but also getting myself set up and situated, sometimes dreading and often crying over it. And then there's the act of feeding your baby, burping them, and rocking them back to sleep. It's not much easier with formula, either. You have to make the bottle and then go through the same steps, plus you'll need to wash and sterilize when you're finished.

According to the Centers for Disease Control and Prevention, a whopping 83.2 percent of us start out breastfeeding our babies. And after speaking with what feels like the majority of that percentage, I can tell you that we all struggle and have challenges of some sort.

I was always ambivalent about my feeding plan. I didn't have strong feelings either way, but I planned to breastfeed because, to be perfectly honest, everyone who treated me throughout my pregnancy approached the subject as if there were no other option. No one discussed formula or gave me brochures about it. It was always—and only—about breastfeeding.

I'm not ashamed to admit that I had no maternal urge to breastfeed my son. I planned to do so because I believed it was best for his health, though I secretly hoped it wouldn't work out and we'd be forced to stop and switch to formula. I suppose I may have actually been planning my exit strategy before we even began.

When I was pregnant, I read articles, blog posts, and books, and I talked to friends. I received information from my ob-gyn, and my husband and I spent four hours in a class with a lactation consultant. We were given baby dolls and a variety of nursing pillows. We practiced holds, learned about pumping and latches, and heard about the myriad benefits breastfeeding provides. And we received warnings about everything that could possibly go wrong, from clogged ducts to mastitis. Sounds thorough, doesn't it? It was. Did it leave me prepared? In a general sense, sure. But in reality, not at all.

It's like learning how to swim by reading books and attending lectures, then practicing in your living room. You can't lie on the floor, kick your legs, and stroke your arms, and suddenly declare that you now know how to swim. It doesn't work like that. You need to actually immerse yourself in a body of water. You can prep all you want and call yourself a swimmer, but the bottom line is you're not—until you jump into that water.

The same goes for breastfeeding.

Any progress I made with it in the hospital didn't translate when I arrived home. In the hospital, I was in a bed that could be adjusted to a perfect angle, and I had nurses and lactation consultants to help; in fact, many times they would actually hold my baby to my breast and I'd just have to sit there. If I had any issues, someone would show up with a quick tip. But at home it was me, my newly massive boobs that were as hard as steel, and a very hungry baby. There is no better way to describe the scene than that of an angry, hungry baby bird, opening his mouth and wailing, waiting for a worm. Except it was my child and he didn't want a worm; he wanted my nipple.

For something as natural as breastfeeding a baby, there was nothing natural about it for me. It wasn't a skill I magically unlocked through maternal instincts; it was awkward and scary. I don't mean to frighten anyone or pretend that my experience is universal. But I know that, for me and others, it's neither easy nor natural. And it's okay if you feel that way. You're not doing anything wrong.

On day three, my son had his first patch of cluster-feedings. During cluster-feeding, your baby may seem hungrier than normal or want to be on the breast continuously for anywhere from thirty minutes to an hour.

The next morning, I was miserable. When my husband asked how much sleep I got and I answered, "None," he replied, "We're all tired." I explained that I wasn't exaggerating, that our baby had been cluster-feeding and I really got no sleep. He looked at me, confused, and said that he had read that it "wasn't a thing." I marched right over to our bookshelf, grabbed the first baby book I could find, and opened it to cluster-feeding. I held it out in his direction and asked, "See?" before I threw it at him. I don't regret it because:

1. I didn't actually hit him.

2. I was exhausted.

3. He was being rude.

4. I was overwhelmed by hormones.

EXPERT TIP

Cluster-feeding is a completely normal phase during growth spurts, milestones, or illness, and any time your baby just needs extra comfort and soothing. It usually occurs around two weeks, three months, six months, and nine months, but it's not always on the dot. All babies are different and may cluster-feed earlier or later, but those are general marks to go by. Cluster-feeding is also one of the best ways to build and establish your milk supply. The basic foundation of breastfeeding is about supply and demand. When more demand is put on your body to make milk, your body will get that signal and respond.

Mothers should be prepared to be tired when cluster-feeding begins but know that it's temporary. Cluster-feeding is a great time to utilize support systems and your partner. They can be the arms and legs while you are camped out on the couch or in a preferred spot with the baby. It's important to stay hydrated, eat plenty of snacks, and sleep whenever possible, so I suggest always having things you constantly reach for within arm's length. I also suggest utilizing baby-wearing during this time because it's a great way to keep the baby close while having free hands, and the baby can even nurse while in a ring sling or carrier.

—Leah Castro

Those first few days were mostly about following a pattern of baby caregiving. My entire purpose in life felt like it had been reduced almost overnight to just two responsibilities: producing milk and breastfeeding. I'd gone into the hospital a confident woman in charge of her own life and emerged a shell of my former self. I had lost control of my bladder, I was peeing and bleeding into diapers, I had an incision across my midsection, every inch of my body was hurting, and I had little to no say in how I spent my day. I was there to feed and care for this baby, period.

I can't say it enough: This time is about survival. You may be tired, yet in a haze of happiness or, as I was, feeling depleted and defeated. A newborn will grow into a baby who can be put on a schedule. Your battered body will heal. The awkwardness of holding or feeding your child will soon become second nature, and you'll actually be able to sit down and enjoy an entire meal or binge-watch your favorite show. But now is not that time. Enjoy the parts you can, cry when you need to, and remind yourself that you just have to get through those early days. I promise you, what is waiting on the other side is so much better.

To me, what was most challenging about the recovery is that it wasn't about *my* recovery at all. It was all about this tiny, new human. Sure, I had medical attention, but I felt like it was all an afterthought. It's amazing when you think how we can endure much less and receive more care than we get as new mothers.

EXPERT TIP

Many (perhaps MOST) new parents struggle with early breast-feeding. One challenge I see is women feel it has to be all or nothing. There isn't enough support for partial breastfeeding. I, too, thought I was failing as I couldn't provide exclusive breast milk for my first baby. That guilt is extreme for many postpartum parents. I think it is essential for a new parent to understand their goals. Why do they want to breastfeed? Is it for the immune properties? Is it because it is cheaper? Is it to bond? All these things can be achieved with non-exclusive breastfeeding. Those who do not want to or cannot give breast milk know that formula companies spend billions of dollars creating their products to be as close to human milk as possible. They aren't breast milk, but they're as close as we can get after decades of research and development. They are safe and healthful options. Fed is best. But it doesn't have to be 100 percent or 0 percent.

Breastfeeding my first baby was the hardest thing I have ever done. Harder than medical school, residency, fellowship, or any other part of parenthood (in my twelve years as a mom so far). It was exhausting and emotionally draining and very, very stressful. I didn't have enough milk. He caused me pain. I pumped and took medication and herbs all day.

—Dina Kulik, MD

After my tonsillectomy, I was sent home to bed where all I had to do was sleep and rest. This time my physical pain was worse and I was more heavily medicated, yet somehow I was expected to take care of a very delicate and needy newborn. It's a little off-balance when you think about it.

Eventually, it did start to hurt less. I was walking around and didn't have to brace my midsection when I moved. My incision healed and the stitches fell out. I could wear clothing along my scar line. I'd say I was somewhat "back to normal" after a few weeks, but, as with any new mother, normal doesn't exist after you give birth.

One final note about this time is that you will find yourself talking about your vagina. A lot. And it will just continue from there. You will meet strangers at the park as you both push your children on the swing, and you will likely discuss the repercussions of childbirth on your vagina before exchanging first names. And speaking of those repercussions, they can range from mild to multiple stitches. You don't have to simply suffer: Those who have come before us have invented things like "padsicles" (a maxi pad chilled in the freezer) and "condsicles" (a condom filled with water and frozen). And yes, I've provided recipes and instructions (see page 306) for you to make both, ideally before your baby arrives.

That's not the only vaginal prep work required. Just as you create a diaper-changing station for your baby, you should set up some postpartum pee and poop essentials for yourself in the bathroom to clean yourself, treat your pain, and likely change your underwear often. And many of these aren't common bathroom supplies. These kits aren't a maybe: You will need these items when you use the bathroom. That said, either use the same bathroom each time or make yourself multiple kits. I've provided you with a recommended list of items for your kit on page 286.

Settling in at home with your new baby is a series of physical and emotional triumphs and trip-ups. My first week home was surreal. We were back in our own environment, and everything looked the same on the surface. But I felt like I was living in a haze and now had a screaming, gnome-looking newborn who rarely wanted to sleep and seemed to be magnetically attached to my breasts for the majority of my waking hours. And the ones when I should have been sleeping, too.

Here's what you need to know: Newborns are a lot less fragile than you think—and so are you. Babies are like an alarm clock that never fails to go off and will loudly let you know the second they need something (and sometimes when they don't). True, they can't speak yet, but they are communicating with you through their cries. Please trust me when I say that you *will* get the hang of this, you *will* feel more comfortable in your new role, and you *won't* be living in this strange postpartum purgatory forever.

Real Mom Story

My daughter was in the NICU the first months of her life. Coming home was a wonderful and bizarre experience.

When we got home, everyone wanted to visit. In addition to my daughter having just left the NICU, it was also cold and flu season. I told my mother-in-law that she couldn't bring a friend of hers along because I'd never met her and didn't feel comfortable having a stranger around. She was less than pleased, but I'm glad I stood my ground.

When people asked to hold or feed the baby, I actually had to teach them how to do these things specific to my daughter because the NICU has its own way of doing things and that's what she was used to. I got so much grief from people about this, and sometimes it ended in an uncomfortable confrontation.

Yes, I was a first-time mom, but I also knew what my baby needed. And if anyone tried to make me feel like I was doing something wrong—simply because it wasn't easy for them or not what they wanted—they were ignored or kept away during that time. I don't regret any of the things I did to protect her, and no other mom should, either.

—Maggie L.

Here are a few more tips to help you get through those first days at home.

1. Make a plan to physically get yourself inside your home.

Your journey home isn't over when you leave the hospital. Do you have to walk up any stairs to get into your house? Will you even be able to, if you had a C-section (which you should always factor into consideration because you don't know what may happen in that delivery room)? Can you walk from your parking space or should you be dropped off at your door? Is there a friend or family member who can meet you there and help you inside while the car is being parked? It may seem like a short journey from whatever form of transportation you use to get home to being inside your actual house, but it can be trickier than you expect. Think it through.

2. Make a cheat sheet.

My mind cycled through the same questions over and over again. Is he breathing? Is he too hot or too cold? Does he need to be changed? When does he need to eat next? What if something goes wrong? I was on the verge of a downward spiral into obsessive fear and needed something to help keep me calm, so I made myself a little cheat sheet, with information pertaining to my biggest fears. I asked Dr. Kulik to share what she sees as the most important information you should be aware of when you arrive home. "I recommend that new parents take a first aid and CPR course before birth," she said. "Rarely is this needed, but it can provide much comfort should this be required. The confidence you gain, knowing you have the skills, is invaluable." She also suggested that you add the following to your cheat sheet to help you feel more confident in those first days:

- Babies should have as many wet diapers a day as they are days old. On day two, they should have at least two wet diapers (pee, poo, or both). On day three, three wet diapers, and so on through the fifth day. After that, there will be *countless* diapers for you to change.

- A baby should be fed every two to three hours, at least eight times daily.

- Babies may sleep many hours a day but should also have some periods of activity and alertness before or after feedings. These moments of wakefulness may last only a few minutes but show that your baby is well hydrated.

- If a baby is lethargic, overly sleepy, increasingly yellow in color, and/or is not feeding well or peeing often enough, parents should contact their pediatrician or go to the nearest emergency room.

3. Make a meal plan for at least the first week.

I can't stress this enough: You need to eat. Don't just assume you'll figure this out when the time comes because by the time you realize you're hungry, no one will have the energy to cook. When friends ask how they can help, food—or even gift cards to services that deliver from local restaurants, like DoorDash or Uber Eats—will always be helpful. Also, you or a friend can set up a meal sign-up calendar on MealTrain.com, and friends and family can schedule and provide meals for you, either by making and delivering them or by giving gift cards. Don't forget to let them know if you have any food restrictions, such as allergies or even preferences. Another option is to make meals toward the end of your third trimester and freeze them, depending on your freezer space, of course.

4. Take advantage of visitors.

People will want to come to your home and see your baby. Sure, they may say they want to visit and see you or check in on you, but that's not entirely true. They want to see and hold the baby. To that I say, let them! (That is, if you are comfortable with the person and want them around during this time.) If someone is holding your child, that means you don't have to. Use that time to do something for yourself. It's perfectly acceptable to excuse yourself and get something to eat or drink, change your clothes, or even—if it's someone you are close with—take a shower. It may seem like everyone is asking to come over during this time, but it tapers off quickly. Benefit from it while you can.

5. Be flexible with your plans and assumptions.

You probably have an idea of how you want or expect things to go when you arrive home, such as where you'll sleep, where the baby will be, how your partner will figure into the equation, and literally every little nuance of your life. That's wonderful, and it's smart to prepare in advance. But you also need to be aware of—and okay with—the fact that things may change. You may have an unplanned C-section and be less mobile when you arrive home than you originally anticipated, or maybe your baby screams endlessly when they are in one room but not any others. Whatever the reason, your home setup may need to be amended. Some women have no problem with this while others find the adjustment upsetting. Also, what works well today may not be the case tomorrow, and you may find yourself needing to change up a routine that seemed to work perfectly fine initially. Things will need to be fluid right now, and that doesn't mean that you are doing anything wrong. Babies are just confusing like that.

6. Tend to your lady parts.

I had a C-section and my vagina was still sore. I can't imagine how much more painful it would have been had that been the exit hole for my baby. Don't disregard that bathroom kit—you *will* need it. Regardless of how the baby eviction took place, you'll be bleeding for quite some time and need to clean yourself frequently. Even an unlabored vagina will feel tender after all that.

63

Take your time in the bathroom, use the peri bottle, make the padsicles, and treat that girl like the queen she is. Just as you are focused on caring for your new baby, you need to do the same for yourself—especially if you had an episiotomy or any tearing. Sure, you can get away with toilet paper if you use it gently, but why would you when you can make things so much more comfortable for yourself? Prioritize your vagina. She deserves it.

7. Breastfeeding is hard and unpredictable.

There are many, *many* factors that influence breastfeeding, and most of us don't have all of them lined up within the first few days. Or weeks, even. Take me as an example. Everyone told me how lucky I was that I produced a strong supply of breast milk and that my son latched on from the get-go without a problem. However, my letdown—a hormonally driven response to nipple stimulation, as well as auditory or visual stimulation (a baby's cry or looking at a baby) that leads to the release of milk into the milk ducts—was so heavy and quick that I was in constant pain as he nursed. I struggled with the various holds or positions, and he would often fall off my nipple because I was constantly rearranging him. Sometimes your production can be low and you have to supplement with formula or donated breast milk. A friend of mine had a baby a few months before her sister gave birth and when it became evident that her sister wasn't producing enough milk, she actually FedExed breast milk to her. Even in the same family, one woman may be an overproducer while the other struggles to produce at all. You can't compare yourself to anyone else. Babies are different, too. Another friend of mine breastfed her first with ease, and her second had nothing but challenges until her pediatrician discovered that she had a tongue-tie, a short band of tissue that tethered her tongue close to the bottom of her mouth and interfered with breastfeeding (a tongue-tie will generally resolve on its own; however, as always, this is something you would discuss with your pediatrician). I will say this until I'm blue in the face, and then I'll probably say it some more: Breastfeeding is hard for almost everyone.

Real Mom Story

I came home from the hospital with a stranger. At least that's what my son felt like at first. When I brought him home, I didn't know what to do other than cry with him. He looked at me, I looked at him, and we cried together. We were both scared, but we grew on each other with time. I think it's important for people to know that just because this is your baby, you are still getting to know each other in a sense and figuring out what to do. It's scary, strange, and overwhelming at the same time. It's okay if you don't instinctively know what to do at every turn. This is hard. Very hard. But always worth it.

—Julia W.

8. You don't owe anyone anything.

The initial days of being home with your newborn are about you, your partner, and your baby. It's not about family and the people in your book club. Or anyone else you know. If someone wants to visit and meet your baby, that's wonderful. However, it doesn't mean they're entitled to get exactly what they want. Of course, if someone has come from out of town or is staying with you, that won't be as easy. But you can be honest and advocate for your needs. Let them know how you're feeling and excuse yourself for some alone time. Or, if you're like me and anything remotely resembling confrontation makes you cringe, tell your partner and let them be the one to explain it to others. You just gave birth and shouldn't be expected to play hostess, *at least* until your uterus stops shedding.

9. You can do this.

Those first few days are filled with a lot of self-doubt. But here's the thing: You will get better at handling the challenging moments and learning to trust yourself. It helps to develop a set of coping skills early on. Don't wait until you can't take it anymore. It's okay to ask someone else to take over so you can take a break. Or put your baby down for a minute and take a few deep breaths. Maybe a cup of tea helps to relax you, or listening to your favorite song. Do whatever you need to pause the situation and reset yourself to a calmer state. It's amazing that you can feel like you're about to lose your cool and suddenly have the strength to keep going just a few minutes later. For me, I need to step outside and take a few deep breaths. Find what helps you and do it. I refuse to lie to you and say it's not that hard. I've experienced plenty of situations that led me to question why I assumed I'd be able to handle motherhood. Then, as those moments passed, I exhaled and moved forward through the chaos, knowing why I did this: because I'm strong and a good mother, the best one for my son. Just as you are for your child.

CHAPTER 4
Settling into Motherhood

This looked much easier on social media.

Besides trying to care for a baby, breastfeed, heal, and do all the other things my new life required, I still had to contend with the torture of the first postpartum poop. I'd had surgery before and remembered that anesthesia can leave you constipated, so after my C-section I assumed I'd be a little, ahem, backed up. Friends had also mentioned that the first postpartum poop wasn't exactly fun, so I expected a little constipation and maybe a small struggle.

It was a lot more of both of those things.

The first few days at home were a blur, and I wasn't thinking beyond my baby, even though I should have taken stock of my own health. If I had, I might have realized that there was one more thing that needed to be expelled from my body. I did the math and realized that I hadn't pooped since the morning of my C-section, which was now seven days ago.

My parents were still staying with us to help out, and my mom, a retired nurse, quickly stocked the fridge with everything we needed for "Operation PE," as she started calling it: operation poop eviction. A quick call to my ob-gyn and we learned that I'd have to stop by her office for some assistance with said eviction if it didn't happen by day ten; my mother was determined to help me avoid that fate.

Prunes, prune juice, fruits, vegetables, bran, suppositories, and stool softener became a big part of my diet. Between the extra liquids I was now drinking to keep up my milk supply, and everything associated with Operation PE, I started to feel like I was floating. I could still barely walk to the bathroom, due to my C-section recovery, yet I needed to pee around the clock. There was more than one occasion when my husband or mom found me crying in the bathroom because I'd peed my pants before making it to the toilet. We decided to ease up on the liquids just a bit.

I really thought day seven was my day. I felt some cramps followed by a few rumbles. I hobbled to the bathroom as quickly as I could, which was painfully slow, and sat on the toilet. And sat. It was becoming a point of concern (and interest) for everyone. I'd emerge from the bathroom to see the hopeful faces of my parents and husband. "Any luck?" one would inevitably ask. "These are not tears of joy," I once sobbed as an answer, before hobbling off in what I hoped seemed like an angry huff, albeit at a snail's pace.

On day eight, I was determined. My most recent dosage of pain medications gave me numb confidence, enough to ignore the dull ache I felt when I attempted to evict that unwanted tenant in my bowels. It turned out to be too much confidence, as I ended up with bleeding hemorrhoids. Don't let anyone ever tell you that motherhood isn't glamorous.

EXPERT TIP

Postpartum bowel movements become a problem if you are in pain and it can't be relieved. The length of time it takes depends on the person and what they are eating—or not eating. Too many simple carbs can add to that constipation, and you may need to adjust your diet. If you are in any way concerned or in pain, please call your doctor. This isn't something you can ignore, because it can lead to pain and, in severe cases, fecal impaction when the rectum is filled with copious amounts of stool.

—Christine Sterling, MD

Day nine arrived and I was convinced the poop had petrified inside me. Maybe it was because I knew I was on the eve of my medical deadline and had no interest in learning how my doctor planned to excavate me, or perhaps my body was ready to explode, but I was finally ready to poop.

It wasn't easy knowing my family was sitting on the couch a few feet away from the bathroom door, all aware of what I was trying to do in there. But, after giving birth and discussing my constipation for days on end, we'd reached a new level of closeness that left me with little modesty. It was painful and I was sure I'd burst open my incision stitches (I didn't), or at least cause my hemorrhoids to bleed (they did), but after sitting there and pushing, it was finally done.

I had tears in my eyes, mostly from pain, but some from relief. I couldn't help myself—I had to look. It was like archaeology, and I was sure I could see the layers of each of the previous nine days. I felt like I'd given birth a second time. Operation PE was finally concluded.

Unfortunately, that day also turned out to be when the backlog of prunes, fiber, and stool softener all kicked in, leaving me with excessive diarrhea. I was so happy to have it all coming out, finally, that I didn't even care. Once I passed this milestone (pun intended), the dread and anxiety didn't end. As it turns out, there would be many, many more things that brought about those same feelings.

As you and your partner try to settle into new parenthood, it may feel overwhelming, like multiple moving parts are heading in opposite directions. But it's actually more manageable than you may think. When you break it all down you can see that everything that's happening during this period of time can essentially be separated into four categories: visitors, your home, feeding your baby, and your feelings. Of course, there is also the whole thing about your baby's health, growth, and development, but you can find that in another book. This book is about YOU.

Visitors are a tricky component of new motherhood: It's a love-hate relationship for a lot of us. On the one hand, you want to show off your baby and have your family and friends enjoy them. But on the other hand, you might feel an urge to encase your child in a protective bubble and issue hazmat suits to any-one who may come within a six-foot radius. Unfortunately, you can't always predict how you'll feel. I assumed I'd want a parade of family coming through our home, but when the time came, I was leaning toward the hazmat-suit option. The reality is that you can't cocoon your child forever, but you also can set boundaries that make you feel better.

When I was about seven and a half months' pregnant, my husband received a job offer we couldn't pass up, and we moved from San Francisco to San Luis Obispo, a small college town on the California coast, more than two hundred miles away from the life we knew. Needless to say, I was not out making new friends during the last six weeks of my pregnancy, and we knew no one in town aside from a polite relationship with our neighbors. I didn't have to contend with visitors the first week home, and it really was a blessing because I don't think I could have handled it.

Living through a pandemic has made many of us more com-fortable with stating our wishes when people come over (take off your shoes, wash your hands, don't come if you have a cold, etc.). But I can remember how only a few years ago my husband was worried that we'd offend people if we asked them to wash their hands before holding our son; luckily, any of those worries were tossed out the window post-Covid. I did keep packets of hand sanitizing wipes in our living room, and I used that as a gentle transition to the handwashing request ("I have hand wipes on the table behind the couch, or you can wash your hands in the kitchen or bathroom").

If you don't feel comfortable setting boundaries for your visitors ahead of time, you can always lie. Yes, lie. If someone is coming by at 4 p.m. and you know you don't have the energy for a long visit, say, "That's great. We'll have until 4:45 or so to visit with you because we have a Zoom with my aunt at 5 p.m."

Remember: No one is coming to see you with bad intentions; they just want to enjoy and celebrate your new baby. However, that doesn't mean you have to be a hostess and let them stay as long as they'd like. You can and should set boundaries.

Your home, specifically how it looks, will be the least of your worries when your baby arrives. As time passes and that newborn fog begins to lift, you might look around and wonder if you slept through an earthquake that upturned everything around you. You didn't. But you weren't focused on cleaning, either.

By the time I noticed my surroundings, there were piles of things everywhere, dishes in the sink, and baby items strewn across several rooms. I was lucky that my parents helped us with household chores while they were visiting, but after they left it became hard to keep up. And we didn't keep up, which was a challenge. And by *challenge,* I mean that it was a big issue *for me.* In my home, everything has a place and I sleep better when it's all in that place. I am not good with laundry and dishes piling up.

I could not let it go, even a little bit. Instead of trying to sleep, I'd clean. I was trying to stick to my pre-baby housekeeping schedule, which was intense, and impossible to maintain with a new baby.

My husband has always been a little more laid-back on that front, so he had no problem ignoring it, as he constantly suggested I try to do. This is not to say he wanted us to live in filth, just that we should take a more relaxed approach. This made me incredibly angry. Instead of recognizing that he was trying to save our sanity, I thought he simply didn't want to help and didn't care that I was making myself crazy trying to keep our home clean.

I'd scrub toilets aggressively and slam cabinet doors. Wash and fold laundry and set it down on the bedroom dresser in a huff. Rage-cleaning became my new pastime, and I did it when my husband was home and could witness it. I somehow thought that if he saw me cleaning and struggling he would feel compelled to jump in. It was a passive-aggressive approach, and a poor one at that.

I suppose I knew this, but I wasn't willing to accept that new moms obviously have less free time than before their baby is born. This means that we have to sacrifice some of the things we once did in that spare time because there will be no more spare time for a while. It's not that you won't ever fold laundry or walk your dog again, just that those things will happen a little differently. Maybe you'll have to let several loads of laundry pile up before you find the time and energy to fold. Dog walks might be shorter or have to be squeezed in between feedings. Instead of trying to fight it, work on accepting that this is how it will be for a while, and that the way you are living now, with a newborn, isn't forever. I eventually let go of some things because I had to. It was impossible to carry on as I had been. I just wish I'd come to that realization sooner.

I also wish my husband and I had sat down during my pregnancy and made a plan for household chores, one where we could meet in the middle with our standards. At the very least, that would have been something tangible to reassure me that even if it wasn't going to happen on my usual schedule, it would still happen.

If you live in an apartment, you might have added stress. A lot of apartment-living moms are anxious about inconveniencing neighbors who may be awakened by the howls of a baby—and how they might react in turn. I can assure you that, for the most part, what you are imagining in your mind will be worse than anything that might happen.

After living in San Luis Obispo for a short time, we actually moved back to San Francisco to an apartment, and our son was a little more than a year old, and teething. I would apologize profusely to our neighbors, who would all tell us, "Don't worry about it!" I assumed they were just being nice and continued to worry. One night, my son bolted awake around 2 a.m. and was inconsolable. After almost an hour of screaming, my husband and I put him in the car and drove around the city for three hours so he would sleep. And so could our neighbors. The next day I told a neighbor what we'd done, and she said, "Please don't ever feel like you need to do that. You have a child—this happens!"

If it makes you feel better, you can let your neighbors know that you'll be bringing a baby home (if they don't know already) and acknowledge the new noise when you see them in the building. But go easy on yourself. Apartment living is what it is, and you are just as entitled to live there with your baby as they are. A friend of mine who also lived in an apartment puts it this way: "Unless they say it to my face, I can't worry about what everyone thinks."

Feeding your baby will continue to be a big part of your life at this time, and you might even find yourself transitioning to a combo feeding plan or stopping breastfeeding entirely— or wanting to do either of those things but feel forced to continue exclusively breastfeeding. Remember that 83.2 percent of moms who start off breastfeeding? That same CDC report tells us that this is the time when those numbers start to go down. At one month, 78.6 percent of babies are receiving any breast milk, which could be exclusive breastfeeding or combo feeding. At six months, that number drops to 55.8 percent of babies receiving any breast milk and only 24.9 percent are exclusively breastfed.

Breastfeeding continued to be a struggle for me, and I was among the moms who wanted to breastfeed less but didn't. Even the thought of it made me anxious. I'd look at the clock

Real Mom Story

I've always been noise-sensitive, so I was more than a little worried about what our neighbors would have to endure with a crying baby in earshot. We would apologize when we would see them in the hall, and we were always met with the same response. They claimed they didn't hear any-thing. I knew they were probably lying, but it made us feel better and a bit more relaxed. They were very gracious, and I think they could see the stress and strain we were carry-ing. One morning, after a tough night of no sleep, I heard a light knock at the door, which frightened me because my husband had returned to work and I was home alone. When I opened the door and didn't see anyone there, I almost closed it slowly so as not to wake a finally sleeping baby, only to catch a glimpse of a cupcake box sitting on the floor of a hallway, with no note attached. None of my neighbors would admit to leaving it, but the fact that some-one had done something for us that was so kind—especially when they probably didn't get any sleep, either—made me feel so supported. And less anxious about the crying, which might have been an even better treat than the cupcakes. Okay, *almost* better than the cupcakes.

—Hailey P.

and tense up, knowing that any minute my son would be ready to eat again. I'd wait for the yelp, take a deep breath, and pick him up. I'd practically have to strip down to my waist, I used two pillows and a footstool just to get into position. I'd look at that little head, far smaller than my engorged breast, and try to psych myself up. And I'm not exaggerating about the boobs. When that milk comes in, yours will look like someone gave you implants while you were asleep, except instead of soft implants they used granite boulders. But that could actually never happen because you won't be asleep long enough in one stretch to undergo any kind of surgery.

My son would latch on and the pain would soar through my body. With each suckle it would start all over again. I'd stifle myself so as not to scream and scare him, and after a few minutes we'd stabilize. He fed every two to three hours *if I was lucky*. Sometimes it was more frequent than that.

One night I was so miserable that my husband decided he would go to the store and buy formula, but we realized we didn't know which kind to buy or how much to give him. For all the information we received on breastfeeding we heard not one thing about formula. Other than a strongly implied sense that we should never use it.

My son was gaining weight, and he was healthy. At his first official pediatrician appointment, I was praised for my magic milk and felt like I had no choice but to continue. I did just

EXPERT TIP

I tell expecting parents to pick out formula before their baby is born, regardless of their feeding plan. If you reach a point when you decide you want to switch or combo-feed, this is not a decision you want to make when you are emotional or in the middle of the night, as often happens. Research the different formulas, educate yourselves, and make a decision before you become sleep deprived. It will be there if you need it and, if you never use it, the formula can always be given away or donated.

—Christine Sterling, MD

that, reluctantly and between secret prayers that I'd be stricken with a deadly sickness that could be cured only through medication that wasn't compatible with breastfeeding. When my rash needed treatment, I even said I didn't mind if I had to stop breastfeeding to take the prednisone. But there was no conflict and I continued on.

Now that I'm more clearheaded and have finished breastfeeding, I see another layer to it that I never recognized before. It's a major factor that can affect a mother's mental health and that doesn't seem to be taken into consideration. We know the benefits of breast milk and breastfeeding for a baby. But it's time we also value how it impacts mothers.

I wish I'd heard more people say that it was okay to stop or change my plans when breastfeeding wasn't working for me emotionally. I outright said that I didn't like it to my son's pediatrician and the lactation consultant I started seeing around month two in an effort to make it better. I explained that I almost recoiled in fear when I held my son because I knew it was coming. Looking back, I even see how my misery fed my depression—or vice versa—and it didn't do my postpartum mental health any favors.

EXPERT TIP

If you do decide to cut back on breastfeeding or wean your baby from the breast entirely, speak with your doctor or your baby's pediatrician about the process or look at online resources like La Leche League. Weaning can be tricky and it's best to do it slowly if you can. If you stop immediately, you may run the risk of an infection like mastitis.

—Christine Sterling, MD

Yes, breastfeeding is great. And we need to tout the benefits and give women as much education as they need. But we also need to reinforce the idea that a baby needs a happy mom *more* than they need the benefits of breast milk. And that sometimes our mental health isn't compatible with breastfeeding.

It's good to breastfeed. It's also good not to. Ultimately, fed is best. And being fed by a mentally healthy and happy mother is even better.

My feelings were all over the place. My husband went back to work after three weeks of being home and I felt a sense of loneliness as never before. I was tied to my son's schedule, which was fine because I knew no one and had nowhere to go, but, again, it prompted that feeling of having no control over my life anymore.

It didn't help that while newborns may be lovely, they don't do much. He wasn't smiling yet—according to the baby book, he couldn't even focus his eyes yet—and he cried. A lot. He had colic, which is common, but also heartbreaking. And, to be honest, annoying. Colicky babies become fussier in the evening and cry through what is called the "witching hour," though that's not a correct term at all. It's more like the witching *hours*. Several of them.

Between the crying, my son's not-yet-developed personality, and the loneliness, I wasn't exactly happy. I was also feeling guilt. Because while I loved my son, I wasn't in love with him. I looked at him and thought he was a sweet little baby that I wanted to cuddle and protect, but I didn't have any overwhelming feelings of love that threatened to bring me to my knees. In fact, when he was born, I didn't even know what to do when I first saw him. I expected tears to pour out of me as I'd seen on-screen. Sobbing until snot rolled down my face as my nose and eyes turned bright pink and swelled. None of that happened. We just stared at each other, and I made that crack about embarrassing him someday.

This continued once we got home and gnawed at me. It started the process of my brain planting seeds of thought that I'd later use against myself. I told myself that I was a bad mom. He deserved better than me. Good moms love their children madly, so I must not be one.

Those feelings actually began for me when I was pregnant. I was excited and I wanted to take care of him. But I wasn't necessarily *in love*. I later spoke with plenty of other moms who went through the same emotions and learned that it's very common, though I didn't know that at the time. I don't remember when it developed into that overwhelming motherly love, but it happened. And it will for you, too.

If you are conflicted about your feelings, remind yourself that others felt this way and it didn't last forever. In fact, there is science behind it, according to Dr. Sterling.

"People like to tell the story that they immediately loved their babies and that is why they take care of them," she explained. "But actually our brain is set to first feel an obligation to take care of and protect our baby, and by doing that we bond with them."

What I was experiencing was a completely normal bonding process; I just didn't know it. And I never learned that until I was conducting research for this book. When Dr. Sterling and

I talked about this nearly six years after I experienced it myself, I began to cry because I finally felt absolved of all the guilt I'd carried for so long. I was thrilled to know that I wasn't the bad or unloving mother I'd thought I was. I was also heartbroken that I'd spent so long thinking that was the case.

Please, don't let this bring you down if you don't experience an immediate bond with your baby. "Bonding takes time, but few people want to admit that," Dr. Sterling says. "Moms actually worry that something is wrong, when in fact they are on a perfectly normal trajectory. It will happen, but it's natural for that to take weeks to months."

Finding your footing with a new baby is hard. It may feel as if the entire foundation your life sits on has shifted, and that's because *it has*. The emotional turmoil doesn't have to be a guarantee, or at least it can be reduced immensely if you have an advance plan in place. There's a lot I wish I had known and done differently.

1. It won't be like this forever, but it may feel that way.

When you are in the midst of the first weeks and months at home with your new baby, it may seem like this complete and total life upheaval is permanent. It's not. Eventually, your baby will start to sleep and adapt to a schedule, and you'll carve out your new normal. But in those hard moments when that feels like an impossibility, just chant your new mantra: *This is for now; this isn't forever.*

Real Mom Story

After the birth of our daughter, I decided to pause my career and become a stay-at-home mom. All my friends were working, and I was home alone all day with a baby who seemed to enjoy taunting me with her screams. The only other person I knew who was in my same situation was my sister-in-law. We weren't close; in fact, she drunkenly told me that she thought I was a terrible match for her brother the night before our wedding. But, eventually, I became so desperate to be around other people during the day that I gave in and invited her and my nephews over for lunch. I told myself that it could actually go well . . . or at the worst I'd at least have an adult conversation. It was actually awful. She pointed out everything she thought was wrong with my house and how I took care of my daughter. I couldn't wait for her to leave. That night as my husband tried his best not to say, "I told you so," I looked online for Mommy & Me classes. I refused to fall into a pit of loneliness, and I knew I had to take action to make that happen. I want new moms to know that it can be easy to lose yourself in the early days of motherhood, but you shouldn't. Join a moms group, take a class. Anything to get you out and among other people.

—Sofia T.

2. This actually *is* about you. Well, second place is about you.

Again, you have to elevate your needs. You are the one who gave birth, it's your hormones that are jumping all over the place, andyou might even be feeding your baby with your body. Give yourself credit for all you've done and are doing and take what you need right now—an extra nap, food delivery, or help folding the laundry.

3. Put on blinders when it comes to your home.

You can't do it all, and when you come home with your new baby, something will have to give. Everyone in your household needs to eat, sleep, and take showers or baths. Those are non-negotiable. What you can skip, or cut back on, is an aggressive cleaning regimen. It's okay if you wait to vacuum or dust those shelves. There are more important things to take care of right now, and you'll be able to tackle all of that soon enough.

4. Sleep when the baby sleeps, shower when the baby showers, and cry when the baby cries.

When my son would actually sleep, I looked at that as my time to get things done. Looking back, I honestly can't tell you what that meant. Cleaning and laundry? Probably. But, as I said, I can't remember. What I do remember is that I was absolutely exhausted all the time. I wish I had taken advantage of his naps to get some sleep for myself, even though hearing this advice at the time felt impossible. It wasn't. I was just convinced that I had to always be doing something.

5. There is a high likelihood you will pee your pants. And cry when you poop.

There will be a lot of pee, poop, and diapers, and not just from your baby. You might pee your pants—that is perfectly normal. In fact, you'll be in great company—most women I know had some form of bladder leakage. Laugh, let it go, and clean it up. And that first postpartum poop will likely hurt. But, I promise, you will not rip your anus, no matter how much it feels like that might happen.

6. There's no way to sugarcoat this: It's going to suck at times.

There will be difficult moments, both emotionally and physically. But you've done the hard part: You endured pregnancy and having an entire human evacuated from your body. Just remind yourself that it gets better. Your baby will grow and start to sleep longer. They will eventually smile at you, giggle, and say, "I love you, Mommy." This, too, shall pass.

7. Your baby will cry. Even if you share walls with a neighbor.

Babies cry—that's a fact. And if you try to stop that from happening in an effort to mitigate any potential inconvenience it may cause your neighbors, you'll just make yourself crazy. Most people will understand, and most likely you'll be thinking about it much more than they are.

8. Visitors can visit—*with boundaries.*

Anyone who wants to see you and your new baby is coming from a place of love. But that doesn't mean you have to play hostess, nor is this a party. You need to be comfortable and make your needs known when it comes to things like hand-washing, shoe-wearing, and length of visit. Either that or lie to get them out of your home.

9. You might feel isolated.

It is very easy to feel like you're alone on an island. You might be staying close to home because of your baby's constant need to eat, sleep, or have a diaper change. That's not to say you'll never leave the house, but you also won't be as spontaneous as you once were, and any outings won't last as long. Your part-ner may return to work before you do, and you'll be left with a helpless baby who isn't the best conversationalist. I was lonely and craved adult interaction. I'd make up a reason to go to the grocery store and would talk the cashier's ear off just because I needed someone to engage with. Try to get out as much as you can. Maybe you and your partner go out to eat once a week, with or without your baby, depending on your childcare situation. Or leave your baby with your partner and see friends. Do whatever you can do to stay connected with the world outside your home.

10. Bonding doesn't always happen immediately.

If you don't feel immediately drawn to your baby like a magnet, don't worry. And I hope you won't feel compelled to lie or pretend that you do. This is one of those things that no one talks about, but we should. I carried guilt about this for almost six years and I didn't need to. Our brains are not wired to bond immediately. Loving and protecting someone doesn't necessarily mean that you immediately have an impenetrable bond, but you will eventually.

CHAPTER 5

Adjusting to Parenthood
with Your Partner

Spoiler alert: Babies are not good for relationships.

My son was just shy of three months old on the day I decided to leave my husband. Archie was in his bassinet beside me while I was googling furiously. He was crying—actually, screaming. Not because his home life was about to implode; he obviously had no clue about that. But because that's what babies do sometimes. Even though he was fed, had a dry diaper, and I had just held him for almost two hours while he slept, he screamed.

He eventually stopped, but I was nowhere near finished with my online search. I was looking at apartment rentals, divorce attorneys, and how marital property is split in the state of California once the union is dissolved. Yes, I was tired and frantic; my searches were a bit erratic and followed no linear path. But I wasn't being dramatic or exaggerating my feelings. I was finished and wanted out.

Our marriage was falling apart because of everything. And nothing. Everything, as in the big blowout fights that we'd been having since our son was born. Anytime we had to discuss something that required an opinion, we seemed to skip 0 through 9 and instead began the conversation at 10. It could be as simple as what we wanted to eat for dinner, but tensions were so high that going into any conversation felt like someone was ringing a bell, signaling the start of a new round in a boxing match.

And it was also nothing. Sometimes there were no arguments and no issues that I could put my finger on, but everything felt off. My husband had begun to feel like a stranger. We didn't laugh together. All we ever talked about was our son, and I found myself not even enjoying being around him.

We'd just had yet another fight on the phone when he'd called me from work to check in. I can't even remember what it was about because it was so insignificant. Maybe I asked him to pick up baby wipes on his way home or he told me he felt tired that day. It didn't matter because *everything* was a trigger for us at that point.

It was the moment when I felt like I'd finally had enough. The best thing for everyone was to end this now and somehow salvage enough goodwill that we could be amicable co-parents. But, based on the way things had been going, even that seemed like an unlikely possibility.

What I didn't know at the time was that it wasn't just us. A newborn can—and likely will—strain any relationship to varying degrees. It doesn't matter how long you've been together or if you rarely have conflicts or disagreements: Once you become parents, everything will change.

"For around thirty years, researchers have studied how having children affects a marriage, and the results are conclusive:

The relationship between spouses suffers once kids come along," says Matthew D. Johnson, PhD, professor of psychology at Binghamton University and author of *Great Myths of Intimate Relationships: Dating, Sex, and Marriage.* "Comparing couples with and without children, researchers found that the rate of the decline in relationship satisfaction is nearly twice as steep for couples who have children as it is for childless couples. In the event that a pregnancy is unplanned, the parents experience even greater negative impacts on their relationship."

There's not one specific reason this happens, but a lot of it boils down to communication. Or rather a lack thereof. Most of us don't enter into parenthood with a specific plan of how we'll work with our partner. We learn what to do with our babies and our bodies but assume the rest of it will work itself out. There are no advance conversations about things like who will handle which task; this can result in one parent thinking that they do the bulk of the work and feeling unsupported. But without asking directly for what we need, our partner may not know what to give, compounding the cycle. Suddenly, we've created a series of unrealistic expectations for one another, and if it's not resolved, our anger and resentment only grow.

This doesn't mean things will go downhill and stay that way forever. Once your relationship has progressed beyond the initial shock and adjustment of new parenthood, things may begin to settle down. Many moms—myself included—have noted

Real Mom Story

One day my wife kicked me out of the room late at night and reminded me, for the millionth time, that she could help, too. She was successful, but I just rarely gave her the chance. We knew what the other needed (most times) in our child-free life, but now everything was different. I would get mad when she wasn't doing things to help or when she didn't immediately know what needed to be done, so I'd end up frustrated and just take care of things myself. I hated the way she washed bottles and pump parts, so, instead of showing her the way I preferred or letting it go entirely, I did it.

My wife wasn't perfect, either. She would sleep in the basement on weekends in order to get a "good night's sleep" and not take into consideration that I was then left alone to do everything. I don't mind getting up to help the baby in the middle of the night, but I liked her being there with me, so I didn't feel alone. It took ages for me to actually say that to her.

It's interesting: So many people thought we'd avoid this pitfall of new parenting as two women, but it just goes to show that relationship struggles with a newborn are universal. This *will* happen. Be prepared and communicate.

—Rachel T.

that while the problems don't magically disappear one day, that doesn't mean you won't be able to reconnect and move forward together. But you'll have to put in some work to get there.

Looking back, I don't think my husband and I did anything wrong when it came to preparing as a couple for our son's arrival. We just didn't do anything, period. We didn't realize that we needed to, and none of the couples we knew with children ever stressed the importance of it, either. Not knowing that this could happen—and especially that it's quite common—made it all the worse. I thought it was something specific to our marriage alone.

My husband and I prepared with all the gear, we intellectually prepared by learning infant CPR, but we never readied ourselves for how we would handle being parents *together*. In the years since my son was born, I've spoken with many moms who impart the necessity of partners breaking down parenting duties not only before your baby is born, but many suggest discussing it even before you become pregnant. It may sound like overkill, but I can guarantee you that no one wants to be two weeks deep into new motherhood only to learn that your co-parent has no intention of helping with night wakings.

There is no topic that you should shy away from talking about when it comes to preparing for parenthood. Talk through it all—yes, even that awkward chat about his overbearing mother—before bringing your baby home. I've provided an extensive list of items to discuss before you are in the trenches of new parenthood (page 288). Ensuring that you are aligned with one another ahead of time can save you from a lot of confusion, fighting, and resentment later on.

> **A note:** *We weren't miserable every moment of each day. However, no one wants to read an entire chapter about how my husband and I spent that time cocooned in a love bubble while our precious newborn pooped rainbows. There's nothing to learn from that. Instead, I am going to focus on the hard parts and the wisdom we'd gained by the time we reached the other side.*
>
> *I am making a point to clarify this because I can only imagine that some people will read this chapter and think,* They have a terrible marriage, my relationship is nothing like that. We're a strong couple, nothing like this will happen to us, *and dismiss everything they will read in the following pages. We also considered ourselves a strong couple, and we are. We were back then as well. And that is exactly what I am trying to tell you: Having a baby will test any relationship. Please don't read this and write it off as only problems "other people" have—which is exactly what I might have done had I been reading this during my pregnancy.*

The disconnect started for me in the hospital. My husband was exhausted, as was I, but it seemed to me that he was prioritizing his needs and feelings over mine. I had a C-section and couldn't pick my baby up from the bassinet when he needed to nurse; someone had to hand him to me. And while my husband often filled this role, there were a few times when he wouldn't wake up to do it and I had to resort to calling a nurse to come in as he snoozed. He later told me he heard me, but

---

EXPERT TIP

One of the first things I recommend is working with a couples counselor. There can be many challenges for a new mom when it comes to getting out of the house with a baby and going to therapy, but you have to look at it through a medical lens. If you were physically ill, you'd see a medical doctor. This is no different. It needs to be a priority, and if your schedules don't allow for you to go with your partner, go yourself. It's necessary for new moms to feel a sense of support or have a moderator, and a therapist can do that. If you physically can't go, telehealth is a great option and one that has been very normalized since the pandemic. If there is a financial concern, you can always ask for a sliding scale payment system. The key thing is not to think of therapy as unattainable and that it needs to happen every week. That's difficult to do for most people. Therapy can be once a month or whatever you need to work with your schedule. Many providers are working to make mental health more accessible for everyone.

—Morgan Francis, PsyD,
clinical psychologist and licensed therapist

---

assumed I'd give up and call the nurse to help. It enraged me: Here I'd been sliced open to bring *our* child into the world, yet he couldn't get up to help me so that I could feed him with my massively engorged and painful breasts? He also went home during the day to nap. I was breastfeeding every two hours (at least) and recovering from surgery while he was just trying to squeeze in as much sleep as he could.

What I know now, years later, because we have since discussed it with clear and rested heads, is that he was trying to get as much sleep as possible during those early days because he knew that when we went home we would be on our own. He wanted to take advantage of the help we had in the hospital and sleep so that he would be more coherent—and able to help me—after we left. It was a great plan, actually. Too bad he never told me. And I never asked.

That initial bout of miscommunication was never cleared up and I carried with me the assumptions I made about his intent and let my anger build. I was irritated with him, which he sensed, and he felt that I was unjustly upset with him and he had no idea why. It seems so silly and could have been easily fixed. I assumed that we would find a rhythm within a few days, and that the divide that began growing between us back in the hospital would be temporary. I was wrong.

If it hadn't been so isolating and heartbreaking, it would have been almost comical how we had such completely opposite views on everything. If I wanted A, he was dead set on Z—and that wasn't up for discussion; it was the hill he was willing to die upon. And I was no more flexible. There was no middle ground we could find.

On top of all this, I was also slowly descending into the throes of postpartum depression (page 181), though I didn't realize it at the time, and that clouded everything that came into and out of my brain.

EXPERT TIP

With communication it's not just about what you say but what each of you are hearing. Often, when someone says something, the other person will take it the wrong way and infer a meaning that doesn't exist—not because of anything that was said but because of their own experiences. You need to be aware of this and then look at your underlying belief system—what you think about yourself—to learn why you may be doing this.

—Morgan Francis, PsyD, LPC

By now you are probably wondering how we managed to stay together. I wish I could say that it was something like us sitting down one day and calmly addressing our concerns, but it wasn't. It was a fight, a really big one, that happened the same day I turned to Google.

My husband came home from work for lunch, as he often did, except this day we didn't even touch our food before the conversation turned into an argument. Finally. We must have sat there for almost two hours, sometimes yelling and often crying. We each shared stories of the times over the past few months when we felt attacked by the other person, but the gist of everything we said was always the same. I thought he was always mad and judging every move I made, and he said I seemed to be trying to push him out and do everything by myself.

But we were at last on the path to healing.

It took some time for us to fully get our relationship back on track, but we did. When we finally opened up to each other, we discovered that we actually weren't at opposite ends of every single issue. Rather, we were just two scared and exhausted new parents who internalized our feelings because we didn't want to make a bad situation worse.

Every story has two sides. Here is a breakdown of some of our most acrimonious disputes.

Issue: I thought he was always mad at me.

I said: Anytime we talked, he was quiet and not like himself.

He said: He was scared that he would hold our son incorrectly or do something wrong and injure him. He existed in a state of fear and thought I was judging every move he made as a father. Between that and the exhaustion, he started to shut down.

Issue: He hovered around when I did anything with the baby but didn't want me anywhere near him when he was handling the baby's care.

I said: He didn't trust me and thought I was a bad mom. It both upset and angered me.

He said: He felt like he had no idea what he was doing and was in awe, and a little jealous of what he called my "natural instincts." He wanted to watch me and learn but was also self-conscious when he changed a diaper or did anything with the baby. He worried that I would silently assess his abilities and be upset with how he did things, so he wanted to "practice more" in private.

Issue: I was upset about having visitors coming over to meet the baby.

I said: I started having panic attacks about visitors, convinced that our son would contract RSV (respiratory syncytial virus, a life-threatening viral infection that can cause newborns to develop cold-like symptoms and sometimes pneumonia).

He said: I never explained the extent of the panic attacks, or the specific fears behind them. He only heard me say, "I'm scared of people being around the baby," and with no good explanation of why. He felt I was trying to keep people away, specifically his family. This popped up a few days before we were expecting visitors from—you guessed it—his family. (For the record, my mom sneezed while we were talking on the phone around this time, and I told her to postpone her next planned visit as well.)

Issue: He would come home every day full of unsolicited advice from strangers ("The guy at the dry cleaner was saying we should do this . . .") and it enraged me.

I said: I thought it was yet again another way to tell me I was doing a terrible job as a mother. Obviously, if I were doing things "right," we wouldn't need outside help. Why was he trusting other people—some of them strangers—over me? I felt that all that so-called advice was just throwing gasoline onto an already out-of-control inferno.

He said: He looked at it that people were coming from a good place and just wanted to help. Things obviously weren't perfect, so what would it hurt to try? And if we didn't think the advice sounded good, we could just ignore it entirely, or take parts that we liked and discard the rest.

Issue: I felt like my body was falling apart, yet when I expressed that, or any worry or fear about my new postpartum self, he seemed to dismiss my concerns.

I said: He didn't care about me or anything I was feeling. I was in pain, my healing was slow, and I felt as if I were living in another person's body. On top of that, I was crying all the time.

I just wanted him to listen and acknowledge my fears. Instead, he would tell me I was overreacting.

He said: He agrees that he should have just let me vent, but he felt that everything was falling apart around us and it was up to him to keep things together. He saw me sick, he saw me struggling, and he was afraid that if he encouraged me to "give in to those feelings entirely, things would only get worse," which he said he envisioned as me crawling into bed and never getting out again. He was scrambling to try to keep me going. He said he wasn't dismissing it, he was just attempting to "fix" things by trying to keep my spirits up.

What I neglected to consider were the key truths about all new parents, a list you should memorize or print out and stick on yours and your partner's forehead, so you are reminded of them each time you interact with one another.

1. You are both exhausted, and that is a bigger problem than you may realize. You need to acknowledge what that could be doing to you both.

Sleep deprivation doesn't just mean you are tired; it really and truly will impact you both physically and mentally. It can weaken your immunity; increase your risk of diabetes, high blood pressure, and heart disease; cause you to overeat; kill your libido (but you won't even be cleared for sex by your

Real Mom Story

My husband and I have three kids, and I have told him I want a divorce during the newborn stage with each child. Fatherhood brought out an ugly side of him that I'd never seen before. He started to micromanage everything I did, from taking care of our baby to how I cleaned the house. I guess we just assumed we'd be aligned on things, but we weren't. We didn't agree on rules and discipline, how involved his mother would be, or even whether or not to let the kids have screen time. We've fought and said terrible things to each other, because babies don't fix relationships; they make them harder. If there are small cracks, they will just get bigger. Be on the same page about everything. Don't assume you agree; talk about it.

—Lauren F.

doctor for at least six weeks); and make you more prone to falls. All that aside, it's the mental effects that are going to wreak havoc on your relationship. Your mood changes, possibly making you irritable, emotional, short-tempered, and even anxious or depressed. Concentration, short-term memory, and problem-solving skills may not be up to your usual standards.

2. You were both handed a tiny baby, who came with no instruction manual, and asked to keep it alive—with no prior experience. That's a little scary.

I don't care if you are or were a babysitter, nanny, pediatric health-care worker, or the oldest of fifteen siblings. Holding *your* baby is like nothing else you've ever experienced. And no matter how prepared you may be, you will feel at the very least a flicker of fear as the weight of being wholly responsible for a helpless newborn's life begins to settle in. You are both feeling that, and it can become all-consuming at times. Remember that.

3. You have a natural instinct; your partner might not.

The so-called "maternal instinct" was never anything I noticed, but my husband did. He said that my presence alone seemed to soothe our son, whereas he had to run through his entire bag of tricks before he found one that worked. He saw my interactions as natural and intuitive. While he was glad that I had those skills, he was jealous. And it made him doubt his abilities even more.

4. You can prepare as much as possible but you won't feel like it was enough.

Even though we took classes and read books, I actually received more training to become a waitress. I was better prepared to serve fajitas than to keep a tiny human alive. Parenthood shouldn't be a matter of on-the-job training, but it is. You can take all the classes, put diapers on a baby doll, and earn a master's degree in swaddling, but it won't feel like enough once you are home alone with your baby. This can drastically increase anxiety. Be kind to each other and allow some time to sharpen your skills.

5. You need to be aligned. And stay aligned.

It's important to feel that you are working together; otherwise, things will spiral out of control and it may seem as if you're working against one another. I never would have guessed that a seven-pound baby could drive such a wedge in my relationship, but in hindsight it was easy. Once you added in sleep deprivation, emotions, and my wild hormones, almost every conversation about how to handle something, like letting our son fall asleep in his swing, became a disagreement. You need to discuss all this before your baby is born, when you have clear minds and level heads. And stick to your plan. Together. See page 288 for a list of questions you and your partner need to discuss before your baby is born.

6. You'll both want to solve every problem and may not agree on how to do that.

All parents reach a point of desperation when they become so consumed with trying to find a quick fix to whatever issue is keeping them from sleeping that they'll start searching for a magic cure. Every person will give you a different answer (because every baby is different and there are few "one size fits all" fixes for anything in life), and I wanted to try whatever I could find. My husband, however, was more restrained. What we should have done was set some shopping parameters beforehand, maybe how much we would spend in each category and how long we'd give a so-called miracle cure a chance to work before we moved on to the next one.

7. You need to acknowledge each other.

Parenthood isn't about trophies or awards. But, like anything else, it's nice to be acknowledged when you're doing a good job. After we talked through everything, we then made an effort to say something nice or compliment the other person. It wasn't big, sweeping declarations; it was real life. "Wow, you got that burp out of him quickly. Good job!" Or "Thank you for getting him to sleep. If he had screamed one minute longer, I may have pierced my eardrums with a fork!" We began laughing more, built up one another's confidence, and had fun. After a while, I didn't have to remind myself anymore. It just came naturally. And it still does.

8. You have plenty of time to do this on your own, so please accept help when it's offered.

My husband was of the mindset that he needed to perfect his parenting skills as quickly as possible. He didn't want us to

EXPERT TIP

First of all—and this can be a reality check for many—you need to know that there is no overnight strategy that will fix a relationship during this period; it's going to take time. You need to be talking and communicating with each other about all the ways this is affecting you and commit to making your relationship a priority. Ideally, you could schedule date nights to help reconnect, but that's not always affordable or convenient with a baby. If you can't go on dates, I recommend *dating* your partner. Leave them notes, letting them know you're thinking of them through positive affirmations. Take walks together with your baby in a stroller. Or just sit down together when your baby is asleep and really talk and connect, instead of doing one of the endless tasks that may pull your focus. Making time for each other is a big part of what will help you through this.

—Morgan Francis, PsyD

accept much help or give each other breaks. He thought we needed to be doing everything ourselves and master every task as soon as we could. Sure, we needed to be present and active and learn what we were doing. But parenting isn't a race. Doing everything ourselves just made us more tired, not parenting experts.

9. Relationship struggles are not unique to you and won't last forever.

No one told me that after their baby was born, things got so bad in their relationship that they thought they might want a divorce. I thought it was just me, only us. That welcoming a new baby into their home did nothing other than increase the love. Well, I'm here to tell you that's not how it was for me, or the countless other couples I've spoken with. Yours is not the only partnership feeling the strain. It's okay to be mad and resentful, to be hurt and even cry. Because this massive change will take adjustments, and there will be growing pains as you make room for your newest family member.

10. Once again, don't forget your place.

This is something I say all the time, and people either love it or loathe it. I'll be honest: It's usually men who have a knee-jerk reaction and don't bother trying to understand what I'm saying. But you each need to know your place during those early days, and yours is going to be higher on the list than your partner's. Now I don't mean that you should sit on a tuffet and have your grapes peeled; it's not like that. But you have just given birth. Your body is in recovery, your hormones are dancing, your breasts are throbbing whether you breastfeed or not. You deserve some extra help and to have your needs prioritized. That doesn't mean your partner gets kicked to the curb—they matter, too. You just matter a little bit more right now. And you both need to be aware of that. This was another area my husband had strong feelings about even though I couldn't see that through my anger. I'll let him tell you in his words: "Think of it like this. . . . Your baby is an airplane, and your partner is the pilot. You're a passenger. Unfortunately, all of the flight crew called in sick that day. Do you want the pilot to leave the cockpit to serve you food, drinks, and make sure you have headphones? Or can you forgo all that for a bit, allowing the pilot to focus on the airplane and ensure a safe landing? Let her fly the plane; she needs to focus on the baby. Do what you can to help her. Or, at the very least, don't expect to be served a meal during the flight."

CHAPTER 6

Prioritizing Sleep

Pulling an all-nighter, but with sore nipples.

I peed in one of my son's diapers, and I also peed my pants. I army-crawled across my son's nursery floor. I paced the aisles of a Boeing 777 for two hours straight, never stopping once. I slept on the floor beside my son's crib. I sat in my car in a grocery store parking lot for so long that a security guard told me to move or my car would be towed. And my husband and I once spent the hours between 2 a.m. and 5 a.m. driving back and forth across the Golden Gate Bridge (forgetting about the toll fee until the bill arrived a few weeks later).

These are just some of the things I've done not to wake up my sleeping baby.

I've spent countless hours forcing myself to stay awake and perform these acts so that he could continue to sleep. Otherwise, any chance of rest would be out of the question for anyone else.

You've probably heard that life with a newborn baby is "exhausting," because people say it all the time. But what does that mean, actually? I've considered myself exhausted before; we all have at one point or another. Maybe you pulled an all-nighter studying for a test or preparing for a work presentation. Or you had to be at the airport at some ungodly hour to catch a flight. And many of us have simply stayed out far too late when we had to be up far too early the next morning. Yes, we've been tired. Exhausted, even. Is that what it feels like when you have a newborn?

The answer is no. Not even close. On those other occasions, you might have upped your caffeine intake to survive the day and retreated to your bed as soon as possible to sleep for a long stretch of time. Maybe it took a day or so to recover, but you were soon well rested and back to feeling like your normal self. With a newborn, it will take months, possibly up to a year (or more) to start feeling human again.

A friend of mine learned that she was pregnant a few months after my son was born, and she asked me to tell her honestly about the sleep deprivation. This was before I had adopted my current approach of talking about motherhood with raw honesty, and I hesitated to tell her the truth. She persisted, and eventually I sent her an email explaining how I felt. This is what it said:

I suppose, if you wanted to, you could try and prepare somewhat. Start by staying up all night. Not once or twice—anyone can survive a few nights without sleep. Do it for a week so that you are truly exhausted, to the point where you forget how to open the refrigerator, then go to sleep and set an alarm to go off 45 minutes later, preferably with a scream. Next, get up and try to rock that screaming alarm back to sleep. Throw in some weights ranging from 7 to 20 lbs. to make it more authentic and, if you can, find weights that squirm and scratch your face (with fingernails that you forgot to trim because YOU ARE SO TIRED). Once you get the alarm asleep, you can go back to bed. For another 45 minutes. Then wake up and attach a vacuum hose to your nipple for the next five hours (bonus points if you scratch them raw with sandpaper beforehand). This is called cluster-feeding and it will be your new nemesis. Once that's done, it's time to get up for the day. Congratulations. You've survived one day of new mom sleep deprivation.

I have medication that causes less of a reaction than my lack of sleep did, and it actually came with a warning label not to operate heavy machinery or drive a car. But being responsible for keeping a baby alive on little to no sleep? There's no warning for that.

My son had hardly any interest in his bassinet or crib. When he slept, it was always anywhere other than those two places: in someone's arms, the car, his stroller, a baby carrier, or on the exam table during a checkup with his pediatrician. I should have just let him sleep in any of those places, but I didn't. I wanted to, but when I'd mention it to almost anyone, the unsolicited advice came rolling in. People have strong feelings about how other people's babies sleep and like to tell you that you will spoil them if they sleep longer than a few minutes anywhere other than in their crib or bassinet.

EXPERT TIP

Many parents worry about potentially establishing bad habits the minute their baby comes out of the birth canal, but parents don't need to worry about creating bad sleep habits during the first two months. And while your baby isn't yet ready for a schedule at this stage, you can start to expose them to some of the healthy sleep habits that will help down the road.

A good place to start is by following the same bedtime routine each night—for example, give your baby a bath, a feeding, and read them a book before you put them down to sleep. Don't be concerned if they don't go to sleep when you put them down; you are just setting the stage for what will become their routine. Stick with a consistent schedule around sleep.

You can also create a clear difference between day and night, which will be something else they will begin to distinguish themselves after about six weeks. For example, when they are awake during the day, be active and lively, keep your home bright, or even have the radio on. And during the night, make your baby's awake time more mellow or relaxed. Dim lights and quiet, soothing voices help accomplish this.

—Kerrin Edmonds, certified infant and
child sleep consultant

My lactation consultant told me about a client who let her baby sleep in their swing a few times, which quickly evolved into her baby refusing to sleep anywhere but that swing. In fact, when they took a vacation to Europe, they boxed up their swing and took it along for the trip, paying the airline a $150 "oversize luggage" fee. Each way.

And a family friend knew a couple who eventually divorced because the wife "gave in" to co-sleeping with their baby, and the child would never sleep alone again. The husband ended up in the guest room, and their marriage couldn't be repaired.

In short, the world doesn't want you to indulge your baby in their sleep preferences. They want you to have your baby sleep the way they think is best. However, they aren't the ones in your house at 3 a.m. And until they offer to come over and stand in for you during those long stretches of sleep deprivation, their opinions don't matter.

There are some things that can't be fixed because they're not broken—just miserable. Like cluster-feedings, and the fact that a baby's stomach is so small that they are physically unable to sleep through the night because they need to eat. Or sleep regressions, which usually last a few weeks, when even the best sleepers have problems falling or staying asleep. These can be caused by anything from teething, a routine change (maybe your baby just started day care), a growth spurt, illness, or anything else that causes a disruption to your baby. It can be hard to pin a timeline on a sleep regression, because it depends on how long it takes for the disturbance to pass. But there are things you can do and know to make the process easier.

New parents are indoctrinated by society to believe that they will ruin their babies by allowing them to fall asleep using any methods outside the norm. But if the only way your baby will sleep is in the arms of your aunt Karen while a foghorn blows, I say buy that woman a plane ticket and start building a lighthouse. Do whatever you can to make sure your child is safe and asleep so that you can be rested, too.

People love to tell new moms to "sleep when the baby sleeps." But I couldn't. That was when I did laundry and dishes, caught up on email and texts, and did whatever else I thought needed to be done. As I've said before, now that I'm a few years removed from that stage, I look back and don't remember any of those chores or how my house looked. I remember how miserable I felt because all I wanted to do was sleep.

The laundry will eventually get folded. Or not. It doesn't really matter, and it won't affect your health. But lack of sleep will. You need to value yourself above all those things because you really do matter more than any of them. I understand, though, that this is easier said than done. Life has to continue, no matter how tired we may be. Bills must be paid, dogs need walks, and we have to eat. But sometimes you can ignore one of those tasks in favor of a nap. Please, sleep when the baby sleeps, at least some of the time.

At best, my son would sleep for forty-five-minute stretches. Many nights I'd wake up screaming because he wasn't in my arms and I couldn't remember putting him in his bassinet, leaving me convinced that I'd somehow dropped him on the floor. I never did, thankfully. I always found him safe in his bassinet, regardless of whether I remembered placing him there or not.

One night, I saw green dots dancing on my closet doors. They moved in harmony, and it was actually quite mesmerizing. *I'm watching* Fantasia, I assumed. I sat like that for a few minutes until my husband found me. I asked him how he was projecting "the movie" and he looked at me like I was seeing something that wasn't really there. Which I was.

I was dangerously overtired and hallucinating. I'd lost all my coping skills and was now imagining things. Yet all I heard was "All new moms feel this way. It will get better." I kept waiting for that day, but it never came.

A few days after my personal light show, my son, who was six weeks old at the time, had a checkup with his pediatrician. When I told her about our lack of sleep and all the "advice" I was being given, she said, "I give you permission to ignore everything people are telling you." She told me to let my son sleep where he wanted to sleep, as long as he was safe, and gave me the name of a sleep consultant we could start working with when he was five months old. Many, if not most, pediatricians and sleep coaches recommend waiting until a baby is between four and six months old and able to self-soothe before you begin any type of sleep coaching.

At last, my husband and I weren't in this alone anymore. And there was a timeline in place. I had an actual end date for when this draining stage of new motherhood might reach its conclusion. My son's pediatrician even suggested that after I left her office, I drive around for a while to let my son sleep and promised it wouldn't be like that for the next eighteen years.

I left the appointment and started driving. And driving. My son quickly fell asleep, lulled by the car's movements, and the quiet calm propelled me to keep going. I'd driven forty-five minutes and two towns over when my bladder announced itself, and I realized that I had to make a decision: Pull off the road, find a bathroom, and wake my baby up . . . or what? I knew I didn't want to risk waking him, so I quickly mapped out my "or what" options. I could try to hold it, but my bladder control was virtually nonexistent since I'd given birth, and I was too far from home to even think about trying. I pulled into a strip mall parking lot and parked off to the side, where I had some privacy, leaving the car running so my son wouldn't wake up. I grabbed a few diapers from my diaper bag and cringed, but I knew I had to do it. And I was thankful that I had worn a dress, which made what I did next much easier.

I peed into one of my son's diapers. Three, actually, because an adult's bladder is no match for a baby's diaper. It worked surprisingly well, and I actually had everything else I needed in the diaper bag: wipes, a trash bag, and hand sanitizer. In that moment it all felt like a huge win. My son was currently taking the longest nap of his life and I was still able to problem-solve, something I wasn't sure I would be able to do, given my lack of sleep. Little did I know that wouldn't be the last time I used a baby diaper while on a drive. At least it got easier with practice.

I kept the fact that I did this a secret for years, convinced that people would mock me if they knew. Eventually, I stopped caring and decided to write about it. To my surprise, it turns out that this is common practice among moms. Whether it be to keep a sleeping baby asleep or because there are no available restrooms, sometimes it just makes sense. In fact, even though my son is now potty-trained, I still keep a stash of baby diapers in my car for emergencies.

We made it through the next few months, in part, by keeping our eye on the prize: the sleep consultant. Knowing that help would be arriving soon made the sleepless nights feel a little less endless and somehow easier to endure. We also adopted the "whatever it takes" sleep method, meaning that as long as it was safe, we didn't care how or where our son slept, as long as he slept. If he fell asleep in his swing, I didn't panic. I just made a bed out of couch cushions on the floor and slept beside him. When he fell asleep in the car, he'd stay asleep as long as we didn't take him out of the car seat. No problem:

I'd just keep on driving. It didn't ruin him, and he eventually began sleeping in his crib once we started sleep training.

The first few months of a baby's life are hard on everyone because sleep is elusive and you might feel as if your child will never sleep for long stretches of time, let alone through an entire night. It's important to note that newborns sleep erratically, no matter what you do. They have no concept of day or night, and their little stomachs can't hold much food. Therefore, they are eating on demand and sometimes even cluster-feeding. Sure, some will sleep for longer stretches, but many won't. And you are doing nothing wrong; every baby is different and, yes, other people are dealing with this exact same thing.

While I'm sorry to say that there is no magic trick I can share with you to get your baby to sleep—or help you endure a lack of sleep—there are things you can do to make this time easier. And some things you should know that will make you feel better. I wish I could take you out for a cup of coffee and a good cry while I tell you all these things, but if I had to guess, you'd rather use any free time to sleep, so I wrote it all down instead.

1. It gets better. Soon.

A baby's internal clock, also known as a circadian rhythm, starts to regulate between one and three months of age. This is when rhythms in their sleep-wake cycle will start to develop. However, keep in mind that they are also growing and developing

---

EXPERT TIP

There are times where you absolutely do need to fill your baby's sleep bank because it's become so depleted, and that begins to affect their ability to fall and stay asleep. I recommend this to all families, and especially before starting down the road of formal sleep coaching and training. Many parents decide to sleep-train because they've reached the end of their rope, they've seemingly tried everything, and they're ready to throw in the towel in desperation. And, when they finally do reach their limit, they want to start right away.

But you need to remember that the better-rested a baby is, the better they will sleep. An overly tired baby results in excessive crying and difficulty falling and staying asleep. Instead, if we approach the process prepared and with a plan, it goes much better. Filling up the sleep bank is one of the best things you can do for a tired baby, and to prepare your child for sleep coaching.

—Kerrin Edmonds

---

at an exponential rate, and that can affect their sleep schedule. You might see your baby sticking to a general routine for a few weeks and suddenly it all goes out the window, as with a sleep regression. Literally overnight. Again, this is normal. It sucks, but it's normal.

2. There are apps that will make you feel better.

There is a popular app called the Wonder Weeks, which theorizes that a baby's developmental milestones, or "leaps" as the app calls them, happen on a set schedule. By being aware of the timeline, parents can predict behavior, know when to expect extra crying or fussiness, and learn how to soothe their child through each leap by helping them develop skills and/or interests related to each milestone. There are differing thoughts among doctors about the validity of the Wonder Weeks, and I'm not here to weigh in on that. The extent of my medical training began and ended with a wound care class at Girl Scout camp, so I'm not one to tell you about infant brain development. However, as a mom, I can say that, bogus or not, the Wonder Weeks provided me and many others I know with a lot of comfort. When my son would wake up fussy and unhappy, I'd panic, convinced that something was wrong. I'd check the app (there is also a book on which the app is based, but I'm not going to assign reading homework to a new mom) and nine out of ten times it told me he was in a developmental leap. His behavior would generally match what the app outlined, and it gave me a great sense of comfort to know that he was okay, and I wasn't failing as a mother.

3. The witching hour is real.

Whatever you've heard about this is probably true, that babies get extremely fussy during this time. It's actually a bit of a tease to call this an hour, because it begins anywhere around 4–5 p.m. and can last up until 11 p.m.–midnight. So it's more of a witching half-day. The reasons could be many: The house gets busier around this time as parents or older siblings come home; perhaps babies are overstimulated or just overtired. It can make you feel like you are slowly losing your mind because it seemingly makes no sense. The good news is that it typically lasts for just the first few months of your baby's life.

4. There is no magic product.

If you feel tempted to buy products that claim to promote sleep, you're not alone. The baby sleep industry is actually valued at more than $300 million a year. Yes, parents spend that much money buying anything and everything they think might help, because sleep deprivation is horrible. And as much as we'd like to see our little babies getting the rest they need, we want to sleep ourselves, too. Exhaustion makes you open your wallet; at least it did for me. I'm not entirely sure if the majority of the products I purchased actually worked to help my son sleep, or just made me feel as if I were doing something to help. We tried some doozies along the way. My husband found an app (which wasn't free; I think it was $19.99 to sign up and a $4.99 monthly subscription) that claimed to have more and better sleep sounds than any sound machine, and included a personalized option for your baby. It claimed that a parent's voice

Real Mom Story

There are only so many skills to learn in motherhood and then the rest is instinct. I wish people talked more to new moms about listening to our instincts and less to other people. We were told from the get-go that certain things were just unacceptable, one thing being holding our baby while he slept. "The baby won't learn to self-soothe" and "You'll never get any sleep!" We had six miserable weeks after our baby was born. He would not sleep in a crib or bassinet, despite everything we tried. He wouldn't sleep for more than two hours at any time of the day or night. We all cried!

We finally gave up and thought we'd just try holding him. Lo and behold, he fell asleep, and I held him for about an hour before I laid him down in his bassinet, where he slept for five glorious hours in a row.

We wasted so much time relying on conventional wisdom instead of going with our gut, and now those are six crucial weeks of bonding none of us will ever get back.

—Kacie T.

shushing their baby helped them sleep better than generic white noise from a sound machine, and it could create a sound using your voice. But the final result sounded exactly like our sound machine would have if the batteries were slowly dying. I also tried a nighttime tea that was supposed to turn my breast milk into some sort of magic baby sleep potion, but it just gave me a raging case of diarrhea. And then there was the time I watched an infomercial on the calming power of Himalayan salt lamps and became convinced that one would fix everything. And if one was good, wouldn't more be great? I bought a set of eight salt lamps for about $280 that I figured I could place all over the house. I'm sure you won't be surprised to learn that those didn't work, either. Of course, some things can help, though every baby responds to things in their own way. But beyond the basic sound machine and swaddle sleep sack, there was nothing that jumped out as a game changer. Don't be disappointed if you can't find that one product to make it all better. Chances are, it doesn't exist.

5. Ignore the unicorn tales.

There is always an exception to every rule. *Most* babies don't sleep well, but some do. We call these "unicorn babies." They are perfect and, legend has it, they walk, talk, and can drive a car well before their first birthday. They also poop rainbows. Okay, maybe not that last part, but you get the idea. You will most likely hear tales of a unicorn baby every time you are struggling. The first type of unicorn you'll likely hear of in your mother-hood journey is the sleeping unicorn baby. It can be hard to tune out. Who doesn't want a baby who sleeps and doesn't require potty training? Unicorn babies, like their namesake, are elusive and rare. And also, likely to be fake. So, ignore those stories.

6. Ask for help.

Chapter 7 is all about asking for help, and we'll go into this in more detail there. As it relates to sleep, this is one of the more important areas where you need to call upon the people who want to help you and let them. There are no awards given out for "most exhausted mom," and you don't get bonus points for doing everything on your own. You'll just make yourself miserable because you can't and don't need to take this all on yourself. This doesn't mean that you need a massive gesture to occur, like someone watching your baby while you go to a hotel to sleep through the night—because that is unlikely to happen. Small things help, too. A great starting point is simply the tasks you are performing when your baby sleeps instead of sleeping yourself. What are you doing during that time? Laundry? Housework? Forget all that. All you need to do is sleep, even if it's just an hour a day. Let the housework go until your partner is home to help, or take someone up on their offer to drop off dinner so you don't have to cook. Hand off even one thing you absolutely must do while your baby naps and use that time for some sleep of your own. It may not sound like much, but once you reach this level of exhaustion, anything helps.

7. A sleep consultant can actually help.

Some people hear the term *sleep consultant* (also known as a "sleep coach") and immediately assume you subject your baby to the Cry It Out (CIO) method of sleep training, which many interpret as leaving your child alone to scream until they fall asleep. For starters, CIO is not a form of torture, nor is it the only way to teach your baby good sleep habits. There are many different ways to achieve this. Sure, sleeping is innate, but falling and staying asleep need to be perfected. And a sleep consultant can help. There are many different methods you can use to sleep-train, and you get to choose which feels best for you and your baby. And it's a more affordable approach than people may think. Yes, if you hire someone to come into your home to work with you, that might cost more, but some consultants hold meetings over the phone or through videoconferencing, or could even coach via email. Others aren't a person at all, but an app. Even babies who might start off sleeping okay may still hit sleep regressions, and a consultant can and will help.

8. A sleep consultant is not a wizard.

While working with a sleep consultant can and will transform your baby into a better sleeper, that doesn't mean your child will begin sleeping through the night and never have struggles again. Your baby will still wake up in the middle of the night, sometimes to be fed. A sleep consultant will help a baby

Real Mom Story

Naps were a real struggle for my son. He wouldn't take a nap, no matter what we tried, and he'd just scream. One day I put him in the baby carrier because I needed to do some things around the house, and he actually fell asleep. From then on, I'd put him in the carrier at nap time.

When my mother-in-law learned about this, she gave my husband an earful. She said we were spoiling him, that all babies don't sleep well but parents just get through it. I was crushed and felt like I'd done something wrong. I cut out those baby-wearing naps and we went back to trying to get him to nap in his crib, which didn't work.

After a week without naps, and with the support of my husband, I ignored my mother-in-law and went back to baby-wearing naps. It worked. My son was breastfed, which my mother-in-law also said was a bad idea. When he got a little bigger, he started putting his hand between my breasts during naps for comfort. I know it's petty, but I made sure she knew that, too!

—Maggie W.

learn to fall asleep on their own and fall back asleep on their own, without assistance, when they wake up in the middle of the night.

9. Educate yourself.

There are a number of safe sleep practices that all parents need to know, and they change and evolve through the years as experts learn more. When I was a baby, my parents put me to sleep on my stomach in a crib that was lined with fluffy, overstuffed bumpers and covered me with a blanket—because that was the practice at the time. Yet by the time my son was born, the recommendations had changed entirely. He slept on his back in a bassinet or crib that was stripped of everything except a fitted sheet, and he wore a swaddle sack that kept him warm and restricted his Moro or "startle" reflexes (those jerky newborn movements that could awaken a sleeping baby) and helped him sleep longer.

My husband and I took a class on safe sleep practices and kept books handy for reference. Not only can recommendations change through the years, but they change as your baby grows. For example, that practice of swaddling that keeps your newborn so cozy? You need to stop it as soon as your baby begins to roll over.

CHAPTER 7
Asking for Help

Sorry to break it to you, but there is no village.

My husband has a framed photo of me on his desk that he both loves and loves to laugh at. He says it's a perfect visual description of one of my strongest personality traits: my refusal to ask for help.

He took the picture one day when our son was around six months old and we were preparing to head out to the park. I was waiting outside with our son, and my husband called out from the house to ask if I needed him to carry anything.

"No, I'm good," I told him. "I got it."

It's become known that when I say, "I got it," I usually don't. My husband often finds me trying to do more than I physically should, so he had an idea of what to expect when he emerged from the house. And I did not disappoint.

I was holding our son in my arms, wearing my backpack diaper bag. I had a small cooler bag with snacks over one shoulder, a bag filled with toys and a blanket over the other, the baby carrier and car keys in one hand and a bottle of water in the other. That was when he snapped the photo, which was also right before he took almost everything but our son out of my arms and off my body.

Why do I do this? I don't know, because that's what I always do. I'm sure a therapist would have a theory about me not wanting to burden people, but I think it has more to do with the fact that I lived alone for so long I had no choice but to do everything myself. Either way, this was not an uncommon sight for anyone who knows me. I also refuse to make two trips to the car when carrying in groceries, and I frequently put to use the skills I acquired as a waitress during my college years and carry four plates of food to the table along one outstretched arm.

I say it's a take-charge attitude; my husband calls it a quirky part of my personality. Regardless of what you call it, it has *not* served me well in motherhood because it is impossible for one person to do it all. That needs to be said again: *It is impossible for one person to do it all.*

Apparently, I'm far from alone in this behavior. According to Dr. Alice Boyes, PhD, a clinical psychologist and the author of *The Anxiety Toolkit,* not asking for help when we need it is a common part of our culture today. We tend to do this for fear of being shamed because we need help and are admitting that we can't do it all. Or, we may have a negative expectation of how someone would respond. Sometimes we don't even bother to ask because we assume that we know how they will answer.

"Having support available isn't what's most important. What's most important is whether you actually use your supports," Dr. Boyes says. "People think they shouldn't need help, that they should be able to do everything on their own. Sometimes support is there for us, but we don't use it because we feel awkward about accepting it or feel undeserving."

You can't compare yourself to what you *think* other mothers are doing, because I guarantee you that things are not going swimmingly for them, either. Your life isn't the same as what it was before you gave birth. There is less time and more responsibility. Yes, it would be great if your baby could sit in a swing while you clean toilets or make dinner, but that doesn't always happen. Instead of skipping sleep or trying to ignore the growing pile of dishes in the sink (which you won't be able to do), you need to seek help. People will offer—"Let me know if you need help" is a common refrain. It's not that it's insincere, though neither is it very useful.

But don't worry: You'll have that ubiquitous village to help, right? If only. There is no village, and if you think you can just sit and wait for help to magically manifest, you will be in for disappointment. I'm not saying this with malice; I expected my village, too. Why wouldn't we? For years we've been conditioned to believe that motherhood takes a village (it does), and that every mother is assigned one as soon as she gives birth (she's not).

EXPERT TIP

When we're not coping, we assume we need a radical change to make a difference in our lives. We feel like a bottomless pit that no amount of support can help. And because most people can only provide smaller things, we don't see how their support can help. But those small acts of support actually have a big impact, and multiple small acts add up. You're not limited to seeking help from just one or two people. Every person in your life doesn't have to meet all your needs. Yes, you do need and deserve to have all those needs met—but it can be done by different people.

—Alice Boyes, PhD

The village isn't exactly folklore; it is real. Or rather, it was. Our grandmothers had one, our moms did, too, to a lesser extent. In today's world the village isn't possible, and we have to stop allowing women to depend on it. It's yet another way society throws the entire weight of motherhood back on the moms: "You'll have a village to help!"

The concept of the village is that we can't do it all, and everyone pulls together to help one another. We lessen the burden by sharing the load. When I was in elementary school, my mom didn't work and some of the other moms in our neighborhood didn't, either. That allowed the collective kids to have multiple people we could turn to at any time. If we were playing and someone got hurt and needed a Band-Aid, we'd just run to the nearest house. The same thing went for water and snacks, bathroom breaks, or even money for the ice cream truck. One person wasn't constantly being interrupted every five seconds to help their child.

The moms were also able to do more for one another. For example, our neighbor's kids could play in our backyard with us while their mom ran to the store to get something—and she'd also pick up anything needed by anyone else. See where this is going? It was a group effort. Yes, we were all a part of our individual families, but collectively we built a community. One in which we all worked together. A *village*.

The world is different today. More of us are working moms, which means we aren't at home (or if we are, we are working from home) and unable to be active participants in that village. The entire model is outdated, yet it is still talked about like it's this great program we have at our fingertips, and it's up to us to take advantage of it. This is yet another antiquated mindset that is still thrust upon women today that only leads us to feel that we're failing. *Where is my village? Why does everyone else but me have a village?*

Stop waiting for your village. It's not real and it's never going to show up.

"We live in a hustle culture today, where everyone is busy and gives off the sense that we don't have the mental energy to help others," Dr. Boyes says. "And a lot of help and support is now commercialized, which leaves us feeling like we are adding to someone's burden when we could just outsource our needs."

The guilt is real. I feel that I am bothering someone if I ask them to grab me something at the grocery store when I could instead use DoorDash. It doesn't matter if they're already going; I know it adds another to-do item on a list they are already struggling to complete. I know that I will pay more, and the cost of outsourcing will add up over time, but that matters less to me than the thought of burdening someone else. Even if I can't afford *not* to burden them.

We have to take charge and change the narrative ourselves. We absolutely can find and give the help we all need if we put forth the effort. But it's never going to arrive on our doorsteps; we have to seek it out ourselves.

Remember those hormones we talked about? Those are going to make everything ten times harder, especially when it comes to asking for help, which is what you're going to have to do. You need to be specific with your asks. Your friends and family are still living their lives. That includes going to the grocery store, dry cleaner, and post office, and you can insert yourself into that. Would you be irritated if a friend asked you to grab them some milk or bread when you are next at the store? They won't, either.

It's hard enough to accept help when it's offered, let alone asking for it outright. I could be drowning in the ocean while a shark gnaws on one of my legs, yet if someone asked if I needed assistance, or perhaps a harpoon, I'd cheerily reply, "I got it!"

If that sounds at all relatable, you are in for a shock. Because you absolutely *will* need help and support once your baby is born. And you'll also have to get comfortable asking for it because the offers are often said more as a courtesy than with any actual intention to help. Therefore, it will be up to you to dig down deep and find your voice and let others know exactly what you need.

I know that I say this as if I actually practice what I preach, but it's more like "learn from my mistakes." In the early days, when I desperately needed that elusive motherhood village, I was mute. Only now, years later, am I more comfortable asking for help, and specifically outlining my needs when I do ask. Because while people will always be quick to say, "I'm happy to help!" you will find that saying, "Thank you. Maybe you can watch my baby sometime when I have a doctor's appointment" won't yield any results. Instead, you need to directly outline what you need, such as, "Thank you. Maybe you can watch the baby Tuesday at 3:45 p.m. for about an hour while I have a Pap smear?" Otherwise, you might find yourself with your legs in stirrups as a kind ob-gyn peers into your nether region while you breastfeed. As I did.

We have to create our own support system.

I had to start from scratch when my son was born, because we moved in my third trimester and I didn't know a soul in my new town aside from our neighbors. They were a sweet couple

---

EXPERT TIP

Asking for help takes practice. Recognize that if you ask some-one for help in a way that makes it easy for them to do so, you are more likely to get the support you need. Look at it like a Venn diagram. One circle is what you need, the other is what they can give, and the focus is on what overlaps between the two. You meet in the middle and identify the specific help you need that can be met by what they are able to provide. This isn't just a benefit to you; it also helps their mental health by per-forming an act of kindness. People really want to help because it's affirming to them. Asking for help makes you vulnerable. Vulnerability invites caring. And a way to bring out someone's caring side is to show vulnerability.

—Alice Boyes, PhD

---

and, although they didn't have kids themselves, they made a point to let us know they had nieces and nephews and knew how trying a new baby could be. They constantly reminded us to let them know how they could help.

Being the way that I am, I thanked them profusely and agreed to reach out, though I knew that I never would.

And I never did.

In hindsight, I see how they made it so easy for me, and I wish I had taken up their offers of assistance. I know we were very lucky to live next door to such kind people, and there is a good chance we all have someone in our lives who wants to be of some assistance. People can surprise you. Even then, if my story tells you anything, it's not enough to have someone willing to do things for you. You also need to be able to accept their offer.

When my son was three months old, I signed up for a local Mommy & Me–type class. It was a group of women, all with babies in the same age range, and we'd meet once a week at the local rec center. A retired teacher led our group, and we'd sit around in a circle and talk while our babies did whatever babies do—usually eat, cry, poop, or practice tummy time.

I walked into the class expecting it to be that cliché "first day of the rest of my life"–type scenario, where I'd meet the women who would quickly become my best friends—maybe it would be more like sisters, even—as we watched our children, who would also be best friends, grow up together. We'd help one another along the way, easing that load that was feeling more and more like it was going to crush me with every passing day.

It sounds ideal, doesn't it? It's also completely unrealistic.

As I soon learned, just because we all had babies roughly around the same time, that wouldn't automatically make us fast friends. We had a shared experience in that we were all new moms, but that in itself isn't enough to build a friendship on. We could all sit around and share tips for soothing chafed nipples or commiserate over feeling like our bodies would never truly be ours again. But if we weren't similar enough people to be friends before we became mothers, the commiserating wouldn't be enough to cement a lasting relationship afterward.

Yes, we were all moms but what I neglected to consider was that we all came from different circumstances. I chose to take an evening class and found that I was the only stay-at-home mom in the group. It makes sense: These women were unavailable for the earlier classes because they were working all day. And while I was happy to see them bond over the struggles of selecting the best form of childcare for their family, I felt like I was in the wrong room.

I stumbled through the next few months. I had my husband, and my parents and my closest friends visited when they could. But, outside of those visits, it was just the two of us. And when my husband was at work, it was just me. I spent most days putting my son in the stroller and going for walks or driving to the Starbucks drive-through in the next town over while he slept. I worked on my writing assignments during nap time or when my husband came home from work, but other than that, I was a robot. Take care of the baby, clean the house, do laundry, work, and repeat. There wasn't much left of me in that routine. My husband would encourage me to spend some time alone on the weekends, but I was so desperate for adult company that alone time didn't sound appealing.

Real Mom Story

I didn't ask for any help after my daughter was born; I suppose I just assumed it would be offered. My husband was still a medical resident and his hours were long and unpredictable. My parents and in-laws would visit, but they just wanted to hold the baby. I was the first among my group of friends to have a baby and, to be honest, I don't think any of them realized how much I needed them—and I never asked.

By the time I realized there was no way I could do this all by myself, I didn't know who to turn to or what to say. Would something like, "Hi, I'm failing at motherhood and am probably the only person who can't handle this alone" be a good way to start?

I think it's only due to sheer luck that I made it to the other side of this. I'm currently pregnant again and this time I put a plan into place. We hired a mother's helper who will be in the house watching my toddler while I tend to the baby. And I've asked my parents and in-laws if they can help with things other than the baby when they visit, and they agreed without hesitation. Not everyone will automatically know you need help or think to offer it: You have to sometimes make it happen. I wish I realized that with my first baby. I might have actually enjoyed her first year.

—Colleen W.

My husband did what he could to help, but he also had work. And while he was able to rearrange meetings and cover me when he could, there were still gaps in the schedule when I needed help and he couldn't make it work. Which is how I ended up breastfeeding while my feet were in stirrups at the doctor's office.

I needed help. And I needed to make some friends. The two seemed to be intertwined, yet equally elusive.

I decided to try my luck with another class, this one during the day. Like the previous class, not everyone was a perfect match, but we were all either stay-at-home moms, or moms on extended maternity leave. We were in the same circumstances, all home with our babies. I slowly found myself making connections. I learned that I had to put myself out there more, to be the one to initiate conversations. And if anyone suggested a park playdate outside of class, or meeting for coffee at a kid-friendly location, I went.

In a class of almost thirty women, there were three I eventually became close with. As our friendships grew, we all found it easier asking one another for help, even more so than from other people because we were all in the same trench together. It wasn't easy at first to ask for things. I felt selfish, there was mom guilt ("Am I a bad mom if I leave my baby with someone else so I can get my eyebrows waxed?") and my general anxiety, but I pushed through. It was easier for me to ask these women if anyone was heading to the grocery store and, if so, could they get me some milk, because, unlike with my neighbors, I didn't feel like it was one-sided. They also needed my assistance in the same ways that I needed theirs.

It wasn't the village of my childhood. But it was what I created with the resources I had.

I know that not everyone has maternity leave or is able to take classes and place themselves in situations where they can connect with other moms. I get that. But you can still find people who want to help you, even if it doesn't seem that way. Trust me on this.

Just as I was starting to find a support system of other new moms, my husband came home from work and told me about a great new job opportunity he was contacted about that day. It was a position he couldn't pass up, and before long, we were preparing to say goodbye to the new life we'd just created and move back to San Francisco.

The key difference between this move and the previous one was that we were returning to a city where we'd already lived. We knew the area and had friends there—though none of them had kids. Still, it was better than starting from scratch again.

I immediately signed up for an app to connect with other moms in the area (essentially a dating app, but it's to make mom friends) and joined local mom groups on Facebook. I had to suck it up and ignore all my instincts that told me not to ask for help from friends.

Real Mom Story

My boyfriend and I broke up in my third trimester and he moved several states away, leaving me to give birth as a single mom. Aside from some friends, I was all alone when my son was born. My mom kept saying how she wished she could fly out and help, but she couldn't afford a ticket. She's never been the most maternal, but I figured help was help, and bought her a ticket. She arrived on the day I came home from the hospital and was thrilled to see me and meet her grandson, but exhausted from travel. She asked if she could spend just one night in my bed since I'd be up with the baby anyway.

She slept in the next morning, and every morning of her visit. She didn't want to help as much as she just wanted a free vacation. She asked me to take her sightseeing or go out to eat. She even told me one day that she was bored! I ended up cutting her visit short by telling her that my ex was coming out (he wasn't) and that my apartment wasn't big enough for all of us.

If I were to do it all over again, I would have trusted my gut. I would have declined my mom's offer and pushed myself outside my comfort zone and asked for help before my baby was even born.

—Jen F.

In my dream scenario, I would have discovered that my next-door neighbor was a mom with a baby near my son's age, but life isn't that easy. I had to force myself to attend park meetups arranged by the moms groups or reach out to moms on the app. It really was like dating: You would read a person's profile and connect if you were interested. You could chat from there and set up a meeting. It truly was a mom date, or a mom friend tryout.

I went on many of those mom dates. I met some wonderful women, but as I had learned before, having both a vagina and a baby doesn't make you instant friends. Even though they weren't my perfect match, I'd still meet with some of them at the park or for walks around the neighborhood. It was nice to at least have other moms I could text when I needed to get out of the house. Eventually, I did meet someone who became that ultimate mom BFF I'd hoped to find. She introduced me to her friends, and soon I had my quasi-village. I was able to do things like go to doctors' appointments alone because someone was available to watch my son or drop him off at someone's house for an extended playdate if I was feeling sick and needed sleep—and I did the same in return. I know it may sound exaggerated and excessive to say this, but it truly was life-changing. I was no longer alone on an island; I wasn't trying to do it all anymore.

And when you realize and accept that, the second part of motherhood will begin.

Here are the ten important things to remember as you prepare to build your new postpartum community.

1. Remind yourself that you can't do it all. And that it doesn't mean you're failing.

I don't want to bother anyone and feel like it's some type of character flaw if I can't do something by myself. I fear that it means I'm lazy or taking advantage of people. What I neglected to realize, and what I want every new mom to know, is that there is no one who can do it all. And your baby needs you to ask for help. Yes, your child, because if you try to take it all on yourself, you will fail. And it will be stressful, upsetting, and all sorts of other bad feelings, which you don't deserve. And your baby needs their mom to be happy and mentally healthy.

2. People really do want to help. I promise.

Yes, you will hear a lot of "Let me know if I can help . . ." offers that are vague and may seem insincere, as if the person is simply saying it to be polite. You would be correct in that assumption of some—but not all. Trust your instincts: You'll know the difference between a sincere offer and a disingenuous afterthought. Especially from another mom who knows exactly what you're going through.

3. Start small and play to people's strengths.

Begin with little asks to test the waters. Everyone goes to the grocery store, and you probably know someone with pets or who goes to the same dry cleaner as you. So, instead of starting by asking someone to watch your child for two weeks while you and your partner go on a cruise, maybe try something small and non-urgent, such as "The next time you go to the pet store, can you please pick up something for me?" With practice you'll become more comfortable putting yourself out there. And be strategic: Think about who you are asking and what task may be best for them. If you have a friend who loathes discussing anything pertaining to the body but loves to cook, maybe don't ask them to pick up your hemorrhoid cream on their next outing and instead call on them when you need groceries.

4. Be specific with your asks.

This goes for everyone in your life because no one is a mind reader. Instead of asking your partner to "help with laundry," specify exactly what you need them to do. Fold the baby's laundry, move the wet clothes into the dryer, wash *all* the burp cloths because we're running low, etc. And don't just ask a friend if they can walk your dog "sometime": Be direct and explicit. "Can you take my dog for a quick walk next Thursday afternoon?" Otherwise, you could end up sitting around waiting for the exact help you need to somehow materialize. It won't, unless you make it happen.

5. Make a concerted effort to meet other moms.

In an ideal world, we'd be assigned a prescreened group of mom friends shortly before giving birth. But we're not, and you may have to work to make friends. Don't be afraid to use the free swipe-right-swipe-left app and online communities such as Nextdoor and Facebook; free story-time and community events at local libraries or kid-focused retail stores; and mom support groups that are both informal (meetups at a park) or run by local organizations or medical centers.

6. Be the first to offer.

Some people may be shy or unsure as to how to reach out. If you have another mom you are close with, offer to help her by watching her child or text her when you're at the store to see if she needs anything. Hopefully, as she realizes this is something you're willing to do for her, she will offer you the same in return. And if not? Try the same approach with your other friends or consider making some new ones. I guarantee you will find at least one other person who would enjoy this type of reciprocal friendship.

7. Let visitors help.

There is always a chance that someone will come over to meet your new baby and expect *you* to serve *them*—even though you're the one with battered lady bits. Some visitors actually get

Real Mom Story

You have to find and accept help—it's essential. I started the process before my baby was born by asking the people in my life how it makes them feel when I ask them for help, and their responses were overwhelmingly lovely. They said they felt honored, happy, pleased to help, and that it made them feel good and useful. Hearing that really helped me feel comfortable asking for help when the time came that I needed it. I know not everyone has people they can ask for help immediately, and it's hard with a new baby to think about anything else, but I strongly encourage you to find people and build your network. It doesn't have to be big, but you need your village, and you have to make it yourself. Having support as a new mom makes motherhood not always feel like a constant struggle, and is the key to helping you find joy—and sanity—in it all.

—Karlie C.

it, however, and will want to help you. You absolutely, positively should let them. Even if it's bringing you something from another room so you don't have to get up and walk, take what you can get. My friend's mom came over to give my son a gift shortly after his birth, and not only did she fold laundry, but she also insisted I take a shower or bath while she watched him. She may have remembered from her own experience how hard it was to find time to do things for yourself, or she could have taken one look at my greasy hair and realized I was overdue. Either way, it was wonderful. For some of my friends, I've emptied dishwashers, walked a dog, babysat their older child, and just tried to help in any way. It can be awkward to let others do for you, but one less chore is one less chore.

8. Outsource.

Depending on your budget, if you can hire help for absolutely anything, do it. You are not lazy or a failure; you are trying to survive. Maybe a nanny or a housekeeper isn't in your budget (it wasn't for me), but there are more affordable chores you may be able to pay someone to help with. One mom told me she hired her neighbor's middle school–aged daughter to come over to water her plants.

9. Find and use free, local resources.

Kids are expensive. Luckily, there are wonderful programs and organizations that can help provide free or greatly discounted resources. Just as we struggle to accept help in the form of someone offering to watch our baby when we have an appointment or a friend dropping off dinner, accessing these

programs for food, baby clothing, essentials, and other supplies and equipment can bring up similar feelings. Whether it's
shame or fear of judgment due to the perceived stigma attached
to government assistance programs such as WIC or SNAP,
or organizations like food banks, it can often be a big—and
emotional—step to accept these types of services. I'll tell you
something: I don't judge you, nor would any decent human
being. As the saying goes, "Those who matter don't mind and
those who mind don't matter." Easier said than done, I know.
However, especially given how stressful it can be to accept
this type of help, I am proud of anyone who puts their child's
needs before their pride. I've compiled a list of them for you
in the Resources and Further Reading section on page 310.
No, it's not easy. But remember, these programs exist because
many people need them. Besides, I guarantee you there is no
one you know who isn't accessing services provided by the
government through tax dollars. Public parks? Libraries? Public
schools? Moms just want what's best for their children. And
you are a wonderful mother.

10. Not all help is helpful.

There are offers of help. And then there are offers of "help."
Meaning, it's going to come with strings attached and it's up
to you to decide if the emotional cost of those strings is worth
it. Will you be hearing passive-aggressive comments from this

person for the next five years because they picked up your Target order? Will you have to repay this one favor by doing ten favors for them in the future? Or maybe they will happily step up but require excessive handholding throughout the project. Do you have the time—and patience—for that? It's something to consider.

CHAPTER 8
Your Postpartum Body

Your baby won't be the only one in diapers.

I was standing in my bedroom in front of a full-length mirror while my husband and our new baby waited for me on the porch. We had plans to go for a walk, one of our first outings since becoming parents that didn't involve a pediatrician's appointment.

Discarded clothes were strewn all over the bed and floor. The room felt stifling, I was damp with sweat, and my throat tickled with the threat of the tears I'd been trying so hard to hold back. I looked at the person in the mirror and didn't recognize her. It was like I was wearing a stranger's body. My face was swollen and round, and my body looked like I'd suffered a sunburn; it was bright red and angry. Was it the heat? A rash? Probably a combination of both.

I was less than three weeks postpartum and couldn't find anything to wear that fit. I knew that my body would very likely still look pregnant immediately after I gave birth, but I didn't know the timeline for "bouncing back." I'd seen so many magazine covers with photos of celebrities wearing bikinis and six-inch heels under headlines that said things like,

"Bikini-ready three days after baby!" or "Two weeks after trip-lets, she weighs less now than ever!" After seeing so many of these over the years, I'd come to assume I'd be back to normal, whatever that was, by now.

I turned to my last hope, a pair of jeans I'd ordered online that were far too big for me, yet I'd completely forgotten to return. I pulled them up to my waist and, like everything else I'd tried on before, they weren't even close to fitting.

I started to sweat again, and I heard my husband call out my name as if to say, "Hurry up." I knew we had a short window of time before my son would need to breastfeed again, and since there was no way I'd ever be able to pull that off in public, I had to get dressed now. I stepped into a pair of maternity jeans, the exact category of clothes I was sure I'd never wear again, and walked outside.

I thought I was successful at fighting back tears, but my face felt wet. And hot. I wanted to turn around and run back inside, to peel my skin off and step out of this strange body that I was wearing. It wasn't just the weight; it was everything. My breasts throbbed and muscles I didn't know existed were sore. I was still wearing a large maxi pad and my crotch felt hot, wet, and sticky.

My husband took a picture of me in front of our house, pushing our son in his stroller. It should be a happy photo, a new mom about to embark on her first family outing. But I didn't see that when he showed me the picture. I saw stringy hair, the moon face, the enormous glasses I was wearing to hide my eyes, and breasts that are threatening to burst through the nursing tank that barely fit.

And maternity jeans. I saw those damn maternity jeans. I told him he didn't have to delete the picture, but he wasn't allowed to share it or post it on social media.

What's funny is that earlier today, I looked at this and other photos of me from around this time and my perception is now completely different. I don't think I look like my body was in disarray or that my hair was awful. I actually thought, *Wow, I look young!* I see none of the things I'd imagined in my mind back then.

This is something important to know about this time: You are likely placing pressure and unrealistic expectations on yourself to have a postpartum body that you think is the norm. And you are probably being hard on yourself and seeing things that aren't there or aren't what you perceive them to be. I was so convinced that I looked horrible after my son was born that I would automatically cringe when I looked in the mirror or saw recent photos. It saddens me now because, as I said, when I look at photos from this time, I don't look terrible at all. Sure, there were dark circles, and I could see in my eyes that I was exhausted. But that body that I'd been so busy berating in my mind? What I see now is not even close to what I thought I was seeing back then. I made it all worse in my mind. I just couldn't—or wouldn't—see any good because, overall, I felt as if I'd failed to achieve what I was supposed to: a body that looked like it had never had a baby. I'd been conditioned to believe that was the normal path for women to follow and hated my body for doing something different.

But there is no norm; every one of us has a different body that will recover in its own way. It took me having to go through the entire experience to be able to look back and give myself the grace that I couldn't in the moment. It's physically impossible to give birth and immediately look like you did before you were pregnant. Don't wait for that realization to come because you'll spend a lot of time being miserable, as I was.

It also doesn't help that after countless doctors' visits during your pregnancy, you likely won't see your doctor again for another six weeks, unless you have some complications. Yes, that is as ridiculous as it sounds and potentially dangerous, especially when you consider that the United States has the highest maternal mortality rate (MMR) among developed countries. And, according to the CDC, 40 percent of all maternal deaths from the beginning of pregnancy to the end of the first year after birth occur in the first forty-two days postpartum. Among the contributing factors to these types of deaths are lack of care, lack of patient education and knowledge of warning signs, and a missed or delayed diagnosis. The six-week wait period that's typical for new moms in the US often results in delayed detection and treatment for postpartum-related conditions.

In short, if you think something may be wrong with your body and healing process, whether it's an infection or an episiotomy stitch that has popped out, don't wait six weeks until you see your doctor. Call immediately. I always say that the worst thing they can tell you is that everything is fine, and you don't need treatment. Which isn't so bad at all.

This means that, yes, in the midst of caring for your newborn, you also need to be responsible for your own health and mental well-being and aware of changes in your feelings, behavior, and body.

If you have *any* symptoms, talk to your doctor—your obgyn did *at least* twelve years of higher education so that she could answer your questions. According to Dr. Christine Sterling, these eight symptoms are particularly big red flags that can't be ignored.

Heavy bleeding. Before you are discharged, speak with your doctor about how much bleeding is considered too much. Most doctors advise returning to the hospital if you are bleeding enough to saturate two pads in an hour, though your personal doctor may want you to be more cautious.

Shortness of breath. A mild shortness of breath is common during pregnancy, but it should be resolved after giving birth. If it persists postpartum, it could signal a blood clot in your lungs or a problem with your heart. Even more concerning is shortness of breath that gets worse when you lie down or is accompanied by chest pain, palpitations, or a cough.

Fever above 100.3°F. Some fevers are no big deal; others are very serious. You do not need to determine the seriousness of your fever—that is the job of a trained medical professional. All fevers in the postpartum period warrant a phone call to your doctor.

Headache not relieved by over-the-counter medications. This could be the sign of some seriously high blood pressure and warrants medical evaluation. Preeclampsia, a pregnancy-related condition that often involves high blood pressure, can progress quickly and is considered life-threatening.

Change in vision, seeing stars or spots. Another potential symptom of preeclampsia or elevated blood pressure. This symptom is not normal, or expected, and requires medical evaluation.

New pain in your upper abdomen. This is yet another possible sign of a blood pressure issue or preeclampsia and warrants medical evaluation.

Pain and swelling in your leg. This could be a sign of a blood clot. These frequently occur in just one leg, making one leg more painful and swollen than the other. Blood clots can be life-threatening, particularly if they travel to your lungs.

Postpartum depression. Postpartum depression and anxiety are common. Sometimes, through no fault of your own, these medical conditions progress to suicidal or homicidal thoughts. If you find yourself having these thoughts, it is extremely important for you to tell someone immediately. If you have suicidal ideations, this is considered an absolute emergency and you should call 911 immediately.

A number of other things are likely to occur that aren't serious, just annoying. Are you familiar with postpartum night sweats? I wasn't. I think the best way to explain this bodily change is to tell you my story.

One morning, I awoke from one of those new-parent hour-long sleep sessions and was soaking wet. I don't mean damp; I mean that I took my T-shirt to the sink and was able to wring out the sweat. *Great,* I thought. *Now I have a raging infection on top of everything else.*

I took my temperature and luckily there was no fever, but something was happening, and I called my doctor.

"Oh, honey," she said in a tone that seemed far too casual for discussing this massive infection that was sure to overcome my entire body. "It's the night sweats—postpartum sweats. Your hormones are resetting themselves and your body is sweating out that extra pregnancy fluid. It's normal and should last a few weeks. We must have discussed it, or you read about it?"

I racked my brain trying to remember anything about waking up and feeling like I'd just jumped completely clothed into a pool of my own sweat but couldn't recall anything. That's not to say I hadn't been prepared; it's just that, during pregnancy, you cram a lot of information into your brain in a relatively short amount of time. Some of that was bound to fall by the wayside, and I guess it was one of those details.

Postpartum sweats tend to happen while you sleep, hence the term *night sweats,* and can range from mild to having your partner ask if you peed the bed, as my husband did. Mine were quite heavy. I'd wake up in the middle of the night soaked, but not just me and my clothes; it was the sheets and blankets, too. It would spread over to my husband's side of the bed. And I would be absolutely freezing, like my body was on fire but the clothes were ice cold. I quickly needed to change into something dry and hope my body temperature would regulate enough that I could comfortably sleep for whatever remaining time I had left of that hour break between feedings.

I quickly learned to cover my side of the bed with towels. Two layers, so that when I woke up drenched, I could peel one off and have a dry bed once again. I also kept a second set of pajamas next to the bed so I could change into something dry. I used ice packs and wet washcloths on my face and neck, and I had every fan we owned pointed toward me. I hated how the nape of my neck felt dirty and salty from the sweat, how my hair would go from wet to dry and back again, then hang in clumps when I finally got out of bed.

Even though I had some heavy sweating, it could have been worse. I have a friend who sweated so much that they had to get an entirely new mattress because theirs soaked through with sweat. That visual should give you an idea of how intense the sweating can get. Thankfully, night sweats are temporary and should only last a few weeks, but when it comes to any postpartum symptom that doesn't quite feel right, call your doctor.

There are also physical changes happening in your body and you are likely having an emotional reaction to each one. That's a lot to be dealing with at any time in life, let alone as a new mom. As hard as navigating this aspect of your postpartum life may be, it is incredibly common and there is nothing wrong with feeling this way. Try to remind yourself that your body is powerful. Stop and take stock of what you've just done. You created a human, cared for and protected that little being, and then brought them into the world. That's an enormous accomplishment. Your body adapted to make space for your baby and now it's working to return to its non-pregnant state. Did you have moments when you thought you couldn't do it? I did. But it's as if my body was saying, "Enough of that doubt. We're about to do some amazing things together." And we did.

As you probably inferred from my story at the beginning of this chapter, I didn't acknowledge what my body had done. I was so conditioned to believe that there were physical milestones I should have met by now—such as no longer wearing maternity clothes—and was beating myself up, mentally and emotionally, because I hadn't seemed to reach any of them at all.

"Body grief is real," says Dr. Morgan Francis. "Society puts pressure on women to have these so-called bounce-back bodies after giving birth. The message is that we need to achieve the same look we had prepregnancy as quickly as possible. That's neither normal nor possible for most people. In fact, for a lot of women that will never be attainable again because the process changes your body. And it's normal to grieve for that."

I don't know what led to these expectations exactly, but if I had to guess, it would be a mix of a few things. The images of royals wearing heels and a dress only hours after giving birth. Celebrities on magazine covers wearing a bikini to showcase their trim postpartum body. And the fact that while I saw some of my friends immediately after giving birth and knew that most stomachs didn't automatically deflate, I never realized how the little changes that occur after we give birth—like sweating, bloating, gas, and bleeding—may seem like no big deal on their own but become a massive ball of misery when combined.

What I realize now is that while the two duchesses may have looked happy in heels while holding their new babies, they were probably miserable. We never saw what went into getting them ready for those photos, but it probably took a lot

---

EXPERT TIP

The best thing you can do during this time is not to have any expectations of how your body should look. You can't compare yourself to anyone else because all bodies and birth experiences are different. Society lumps women into the same postpartum category and when we don't meet these expectations, we feel shame and like a failure. As for those celebrity bodies on magazine covers that the media celebrates? It's not realistic for anyone. These people have a team of professionals working with them to achieve that look and photos can be edited. We have been conditioned to believe that thin equals healthy, but that's not true. To be healthy as a new mom, we need to reduce stress, have a support system, be able to get sleep, and be in a positive environment.

—Morgan Francis, PsyD

---

of work. Their leaking breasts were covered with pads and shoved into a nursing bra, some type of shapewear was holding in their midsection, they were wearing a pair of those granny panties that they were bleeding into, and they probably would have traded some of their royal jewels for a pair of comfortable shoes.

It's not attainable because it's not real.

I cringe now when I see articles about "post-baby bikini bodies." After all a woman accomplishes, *that* is what we focus on? It's absolutely disgusting. Honestly, it's as if pregnancy, childbirth, the fourth trimester, and motherhood are down-played because "everyone" has done it. But it's new, different, and unique for each one of us. It's extremely difficult both emotionally and physically.

We should celebrate postpartum women by saying, "You are an amazing warrior; look what you and your body just accomplished!" instead of just nodding an acknowledgment and moving on to the next topic, because childbirth is common. We only seem to cheer for a woman when she can flash six-pack abs soon after giving birth.

I hate that I was never able to enjoy that first family out-ing for what it was: a milestone with our son. Instead, I was focused on the assumption that I should be wearing my pre-pregnancy clothes and couldn't. I loathed myself and felt like a failure. Once again, I found myself asking, *Why is this easier for everyone else but not me?* I couldn't see my strength. All I saw was a failure because I was "still" wearing maternity jeans.

But that's what I didn't know, time and time again. That it wasn't easy for anyone. I just never heard it discussed in detail beyond the fact that my stomach wouldn't be flat immediately after giving birth. Instead, I'd been conditioned to believe that the sheer phenomenon of simply giving birth isn't enough, that women need to give birth, breastfeed, enter a state of severe sleep deprivation, *and* be bikini-ready in under a week. In reality, all we need is to be healthy. To celebrate what our bodies have done, not to question the speed at which they recover. And know this: You are perfect. You are enough. You are exactly as you are supposed to be.

There are also plenty of women who do experience a quick return to their prepregnancy bodies. They aren't starving themselves or defying doctor's orders by working out while bleeding; it's just natural for them. Genetics, hormones, whatever it may be. That is their normal. And guess what? These women are shamed as well. People look at them like they did something criminal in order to look that way.

We can't win. Either way, your body will be questioned.

I know I may be making it seem as if you will undergo some massive physical change after you give birth, like growing a third arm. And while an extra arm would be incredibly helpful for moms, that doesn't happen. Some of the changes are small; in fact, you may be the only person to notice most of them. But together they can feel huge and overwhelming. To make it easier, I'll literally break them down for you from head to toe.

Hair. Sadly, that thick and luscious hair you've been cultivating during your pregnancy won't last forever. According to Dr. Sterling, around four to five months postpartum it will begin to fall out. And it's not hair loss, it's hair *shedding*. Meaning, you're just losing extra hair that was never yours to keep.

Real Mom Story

My body really didn't change much during or after pregnancy. To begin with, I'm pretty tall and have a long torso. My baby had a lot of room to grow, and my bump never got all that big. In fact, when I was in my third trimester, people would be shocked when they learned how far along I was and often would think I was teasing them. After I gave birth, I went home from the hospital with my belly about half the size it was, and then it just kind of disappeared over the next two weeks. I didn't exercise or eat less; it's just what my body did. Everyone asked what my secret was or told me how great I looked, but behind my back they would ask my boyfriend or friends what diet plan I used. Someone even asked if I had a tummy tuck in the delivery room.

I joined a moms group and one day we talked about our postpartum bodies. When it was my turn to share, I said that I struggled with people's reactions to how my body actually didn't change much at all. Another mom in the group then said, "You don't get a say then!" She laughed like it was a joke, but I know she meant it. I'm not bragging or showing off, but I can't change what my body did.

—Susan F.

You won't end up with less hair than you had before you were pregnant; it's just regulating itself. During pregnancy, all that extra estrogen in your body leaves your hair in the growth phase longer than usual, delaying when it enters the next phase of resting and then the final phase of shedding.

With all due respect to science, let me put it this way: When you are pregnant, your hair doesn't fall out as quickly as it normally does, and you suddenly have more hair on your head than ever before. But, after you give birth and your hormones return to their usual levels, your hair will resume its typical patterns of shedding. It will seem like you're losing hair, but you are simply shedding as normal—something that wasn't happening during pregnancy.

Other than it being annoying and having to put up with my husband's insistence on telling me every location where he found strands of my hair (the car, the kitchen sink, inside his suitcase on a business trip), I didn't mind the hair shedding. But many women do, and it can be traumatic for some. "Losing your hair can be emotional," says Dr. Francis. "For many women, it is part of their feminine identity, and the loss of that hair represents their femininity leaving as well. They feel less pleasing to others and insecure."

Do not feel that you are overreacting or being dramatic if your hair loss is bothering you. Continue to remind yourself that this is expected. Your hair is only shedding, not disappearing entirely.

Face. Not only were you susceptible to pregnancy-related skin changes, like those dark splotches called melasma that some of us get on our faces, but there are also potential postpartum changes as well. Hormones, lack of sleep, and the fact that you just had a baby and your body is currently trying to put itself back together all play a part, and these changes will generally resolve on their own. Postpartum acne; dry, sometimes flaky skin; and oily skin are all common. Keep your face clean and drink plenty of water, but if the problem continues beyond what you feel comfortable with, see your doctor or a dermatologist.

Upper torso. As your body was growing and adjusting to make room for your baby during pregnancy, it may have widened. "Your thoracic cavity actually increases," says Dr. Sterling. This isn't necessarily something you'll notice, but if you ever find yourself trying on an article of clothing you once wore with ease prepregnancy, only to find the bodice no longer fits, you're not going crazy. You may have expanded.

Breasts. If you think your breasts are big during pregnancy, wait until you see them postpartum. Once your milk comes in, they will be bigger. Huge. And rock-hard for a few days. I always described mine as granite boulders. Each of my breasts was larger than my son's head in the early days. They will leak, sometimes one will be larger than the other after a feeding, and the difference can be so drastic that you'll look as if you have an implant in one breast while the other is deflated. But, like most things happening at·this point, it won't be forever. As your body adjusts to your nursing and pumping schedule, your milk production will adapt and even out. If you choose not to breastfeed, your breasts will still begin to make milk, but it should dry up in a few weeks. Still, it's important to talk with your doctor or lactation consultant about the process.

Abdomen. What took forty weeks to create can't be undone overnight. You will still look pregnant. Remember, your organs rearranged themselves and your body widened itself while growing that small embryo into a baby. We're all different: There is no timeline we can follow as we recover. You look exactly as you are meant to and that is unique to each of us. After all that stretching, your skin may feel loose. This may resolve itself over time but, for some, the loss of that elasticity is permanent. Any stretch marks that appeared during pregnancy will still be visible but should fade over time. Some women discover what they think are new stretch marks postpartum, only to learn they were actually always there; they just couldn't see them until their belly began to recede. And your linea nigra, that pregnancy dark line that extends from your belly button to your pubic area that's the result of hormonal changes, will also still be present, though that will also fade with time.

Vagina. There will be blood; it can't be avoided. The lochia we talked about will continue heavily with small clots for three to four days followed by four to twelve days of a more moderate flow, eventually transitioning into a lighter flow or spotting that can last for up to six weeks postpartum. This is a typical timeline, though it may vary from woman to woman. I can't tell you how many people seemed surprised to hear that I bled after my C-section. Regardless of the delivery process, your body still needs to get rid of the extra blood and tissue that built up in your uterus during pregnancy.

Your vagina may have episiotomy stiches and be sore. It likely burns when you pee and feels stretched when you poop. Think of it as having gone through a war. It's a true warrior, yes, but it's also a delicate flower and needs to be treated as such. Sit on custom-made ice packs (see page 306 for instructions), spray it with a peri bottle instead of wiping with toilet paper when you pee, and utilize all the other goodies in that postpartum bathroom kit (see page 286).

You won't be cleared by your doctor for sex until around six weeks, but that doesn't necessarily mean you'll even want to. When you feel ready to have sex after giving birth is different for all of us, and I've spoken with enough women to know that this runs the gamut, from being ready the day they left the hospital to never really feeling like they wanted it ever again. The majority, however, were like me: It took a while before my sex life resumed, and even when it did it wasn't regular or all that frequent. But it got there. Eventually.

EXPERT TIP

It's normal for women not to want sex after having a baby. Hormones and sleep deprivation play a part and, physically, the vagina is in a very delicate state. A woman's estrogen levels are lower while breastfeeding and that makes the vagina dry. Sex shouldn't be painful, though, and you need to call your doctor if it is. Ask yourself, *Am I able to enjoy sex?* If the answer is no, that's also a reason to reach out to your ob-gyn.

—Christine Sterling, MD

You might find that your libido is low or nonexistent. Some women are uncomfortable with the changes to their body and don't feel attractive or desired by their partner. And exhaustion doesn't help. In my experience, my desire to use any free time to sleep far outweighed wanting to have sex. If this continues, you can and should speak with your doctor and talk with your partner about how you can meet their intimacy needs in a nonsexual way, such as holding hands or cuddling.

Some women have no dip in their libido, or desire to have sex, and can't wait to get back at it. And, yes, a few of them can't seem to wrap their brains around how anyone could feel differently. Others don't feel ready, but either want to please their partner or feel pressured to do so. I've spoken to people in every situation. No matter where you find yourself, it's important to be aware of your feelings and talk about them. If you sense that a lack of sex is becoming an issue in your relationship, don't wait for it to magically resolve itself. Talk to your partner and be honest about what you do or don't want. Let your doctor know. Whatever the situation you find yourself in, if you don't want or don't feel comfortable having sex, let it be known. And never, ever let anyone pressure you into doing something you don't want. You don't owe anyone a thing, especially not sex. Yes, even your partner.

Feet. I was lucky to avoid overly swollen feet during pregnancy, but my feet ballooned with a vengeance after I gave birth. Swollen feet are common and normal. This can be caused by excess fluids that your body retained during pregnancy or the result of extra fluids you may have received during delivery through an IV. You may also notice some swelling in the legs, ankles, or face, and some women even experience it in the hands and arms. It should even out within a week; drink a lot of water and avoid sodium to help the process along. Make sure your doctor is aware and monitoring the situation, as sometimes that swelling can be an indicator of an underlying condition. My feet were so swollen that my doctor actually considered keeping me in the hospital an extra day to monitor the progress, but the swelling improved enough for me to be discharged.

Your feet may also be bigger and flatter after giving birth. During pregnancy, the hormone relaxin relaxes your muscles, joints, and ligaments so that your body can make room for your growing baby and, later in the pregnancy, prepare for delivery. Relaxin and pregnancy weight gain can lead to your feet flattening and elongating, so don't be surprised if you find yourself shopping for a bigger shoe size postpartum.

When I look back on my feelings about my postpartum body, I'm sad about how I saw myself. I had no patience for what my body had done—and was still doing—and was instead hyper-focused on achieving the impossible: not looking like I'd just had a baby. The worst part of it all was that I wouldn't let anyone take many photos of me because I hated the way I looked and didn't want any permanent reminders. My advice to you is to try to set your feelings aside and get in the picture.

I was looking back at old photos and found one that especially sums up my regret. It is a Halloween photo of my newborn-ish son dressed as Nemo at my husband's company's party. My husband, also in a costume, cuddled him. I wasn't in a costume; I wasn't even in any of the pictures. I'd ordered a costume larger than my usual size and it still didn't fit. It mattered in the moment; as I said, I felt that I needed to be in a bikini two days after giving birth or I'd be deemed a failure by society.

I cried when I was getting ready as I realized I had nothing to wear for a costume and slipped into what was becoming my standard uniform of maternity jeans, nursing tank, and a cardigan to cover my enormous breasts. The dark circles under my eyes were like nothing I'd seen before. I wore a lot of makeup to try to cover them, which seems sad. We had a six-week-old. Everyone knew we'd just had a baby: Why did I think I had to spackle on primer and paint?

As we drove to the party, I continuously pinched the fabric of my tank top as I pulled it away from my body. I was hot and itchy. I was mostly wearing sweats around the house; "real" clothes, no matter how many times I'd had to resort to this exact same outfit in the past month and a half, felt foreign.

I remember how adorable the party was. How nice people were. That my husband changed our son's diaper in a public bathroom for the first time ever that day, and that they both looked so great in their costumes. But I don't remember what I looked like. And I'll never know how I would have looked cuddling my baby in his first Halloween costume, or with my husband's arms around us both.

I wish I'd been in those Halloween photos, and I can never go back and change that.

Please, trust me on this: Get in the picture, take selfies with your baby, capture every moment *with you in it.* You won't care in ten, twenty years what you looked like. You'll just be glad you were in the picture.

I want you to feel strong and powerful because you *are.* However, I also know from my own experience that it's easy to doubt yourself during this time. And, with so many physical and

Real Mom Story

I'm a curvy girl and always embraced my body. But after my daughter was born, I was much bigger than before and couldn't make peace with that. I started wearing frumpy clothes, joined a gym, tried every diet fad I came across, and finally lost the weight. Two years later, my son was born and as soon as my body healed, I went back to my old routine of diet and exercise. One morning I was getting my daughter dressed for preschool. She'd recently gone through a growth spurt, but insisted on keeping some of her favorite dresses. I didn't have time to argue, so I helped her slip it over her head. The dress never made it past her shoulders. "Oh, no!" she said in her sweet little voice. "I guess I need to go on a why-it, wight, Mommy?" She was saying *diet*. I felt deflated. "No, honey," I said as calmly as I could. "You just grew. You're getting to be such a big girl and you are absolutely perfect just the way you are." I decided to try therapy; in fact, I still go. I'm learning to love my body for what it is and not how it looks, and I've completely changed the way I speak and act around my daughter. I didn't stop exercising, because it's healthy, but I did cancel my gym membership. Instead, I go on family walks and bike rides. There is no predicting how you will look after you have your baby. Accept who you've become and stop wasting time chasing who you once were.

—Aki C.

emotional changes happening with your body, you likely won't feel like yourself, either.

The following ten points will help to guide you through this time and, more important, actually help you enjoy it— regardless of what your body may be doing,

1. Your body did something amazing.

Take a moment and think about the magnitude of what your body has just done. It created and developed a baby *and* birthed it. Which also means that you either pushed that baby out of your body through your vagina or had major surgery that included slicing your abdomen open. If you knew someone who had just gone through that, what would you tell them? Probably something along the lines of "Wow, that's unbelievable,, great job. You're a warrior." Right? Well, you deserve to tell yourself the same thing. Just because billions of women have done this before you doesn't mean that it's not a hard and physically taxing process. Give your body a break and let it heal.

2. You won't look the way you expect.

I can't tell you exactly what you will look like after childbirth, but I do know it won't be what you're picturing. Some women will look like they did before they became pregnant because of their genetics. Others, like me, will continue to appear pregnant after giving birth. Even though I was prepared for that, I didn't realize just how pregnant I'd look and how long that would last. But all postpartum bodies look exactly as they are meant to and there is no norm when it comes to how a woman looks after she gives birth.

3. Get in the picture.

Let people take pictures of you with your baby. Take selfies with your baby. These are not images that will be broadcast around the world. You don't even have to look at them right now if you don't want to. But there will come a day when you won't care what your hair looked like, or what you were wearing. You will just want to see yourself holding your baby. If not for yourself now, take them for the future you. I guarantee that she will want to see them.

4. You may not see a doctor for six weeks.

My son had a checkup with his pediatrician a few days after he was born, and then again at one and two months. I didn't see my doctor until six weeks after I gave birth, which is common practice in the United States. Many moms, including myself, think this is a flawed process. A lot can happen in six weeks. Your body is healing, your cervix is closing, and your hormone levels are still changing and regulating. An earlier visit to the doctor wouldn't be such a bad idea, especially if you developed pre-eclampsia during pregnancy, or had an existing health condition prior to having a baby. Unfortunately, most insurance companies don't agree. Please don't let that dissuade you from raising any concerns you have about your recovery. I called my doctor's office with questions about my incision, and I encourage you to prioritize your recovery and do the same if you think something isn't healing right or if you have any questions.

5. Remember to take care of yourself.

You will likely be wholly focused on your baby, which is completely natural. But you still have to prioritize yourself, at least somewhat. Go to a store alone, have your hair cut and styled, or even take one hour away from your baby to be by yourself and stare at the ceiling. Whatever feels like a break or refreshes you, big or small. It's far too easy for moms to put themselves and their needs last, which isn't healthy. You also need to prioritize eating, which can be a hard concept for some people to grasp, given the societal pressure put upon women to look a certain way, especially postpartum. "When our body doesn't meet these unrealistic expectations, we feel shame and failure," says Dr. Francis. "Instead of blaming society, we blame our bodies and internalize the shame. This often leads to taking action like cosmetic surgery enhancements or a diet with calorie restrictions." She points out that we are all emotional eaters, and that the term is a positive thing. "As babies, we eat our first foods while cradled in the arms of a caregiver, whether that

EXPERT TIP

Many postpartum women restrict their calories to lose weight or just don't take the time for themselves to have a proper meal. Mealtimes should actually be calm, peaceful, and free of distractions. If they aren't, cortisol levels can increase, leading to stress, and food isn't properly digested.

The foods new moms eat are either a room-temperature prepackaged snack or meal, or something cold, like a smoothie or a salad, because it's convenient. Warm food is comforting, and the process of eating it takes longer because it usually requires the use of a fork. Eating a meal in this way allows us to move into the parasympathetic nervous system. Your heart rate, body temperature, and blood pressure normalize.

I tell new moms to prioritize one meal a day—ideally it would be all meals, but we need to be realistic—to allow themselves to feel the comfort and warmness of their food in a peaceful setting. Try this when your baby naps or after they are down for the night. It will help you to feel nourished and remind you that your relationship with food is important. Through this, you can reestablish body respect and body trust. It's actually a form of self-compassion and can also help you avoid calorie restriction and binge eating.

—Morgan Francis, PsyD

be through the breast or a bottle. Food is presented in a loving position while our body releases oxytocin to help with bonding. We are essentially born emotional eaters and there is no shame in eating with our emotions." This means that if you are restricting your food intake, you are depriving yourself of this emotion, and it will more likely lead to you bingeing on food instead of losing weight. Dr. Francis explains it as giving ourselves permission to honor what our bodies need, which is food, in this case. "If you need to go to the bathroom, you don't stop your body from doing that. It should be the same with eating."

6. It's common to skip showers.

There are some people who can't function without a daily shower and make it happen no matter what, and others who don't feel that same drive. With a new baby, something has to give and, for me and a lot of other moms, that's the daily shower. Or the every-other-day shower. There is nothing wrong with this, and you are in good company. Besides, this is what dry shampoo, baby wipes, washcloths, and vaginal wipes were made for.

7. There may be many strange changes happening to your body.

Your hair will shed, your skin may break out, and your vagina may dry up. None of this is particularly fun, but it is all a normal part of the postpartum process. It is important to remember, however, that even if something that has been described as

Becky Vieira

"normal" is going on and it somehow doesn't feel right to you, you need to call your doctor. You can't ignore your needs or put your health aside because you had a baby. You matter, too.

8. Don't be swayed by a so-called miracle product.

Your social media will become inundated with sponsored posts trying to sell you something *revolutionary* that will help you to get back the pre-baby body that you lost. Let me tell you something: You didn't lose anything. You won't get that body back because it no longer exists. You have changed and evolved since giving birth, and so has your body. It's a force of nature that just did something fantastic. Why would you want to regress now? These promises will come in the form of pills, powdered shakes, workout programs, gummies, paid subscriptions—you name it. But they aren't miraculous and can't be a one-size-fits-all treatment because we are all different and our bodies need different things. You don't need these things: What new moms need is to be seen, heard, and helped. It's easy to be tempted—I've been there myself. And these companies and salespeople know what they're doing; they will sound convincing, especially when you are in a vulnerable state.

Dr. Francis explains it well: "Information reduces anxiety. So when we are anxious about our current state, we look for something to guide us. If you're on an airplane and there is turbulence, you want the pilot to come on and tell you what's

Real Mom Story

I still looked pregnant after my son was born, as most women do. I can't say I loved my postpartum body, but I was also so busy that it wasn't a priority. I know now that I was suffering from postpartum depression during that time. In addition to crying all the time and never leaving the house, I stopped eating and began quickly losing weight. Too quickly. I wasn't exercising or eating healthy; I was depressed. My appetite was nonexistent and I had to force myself to sip nutritional smoothies to keep up my energy and maintain my milk supply. My husband thought my sadness and appetite loss was some postpartum quirk that would eventually resolve. He set an alarm on my phone to remind me to eat and filled our house with my favorite foods, but it didn't help. As the pounds fell off, everyone started to praise me because my midsection was flat. People actually said to me, "Keep up the good work with your weight loss!"

What I know now is that dramatic weight loss can be a sign of depression. If you know a new mom who suddenly loses a lot of weight without even trying, please check in with her. You might be the reason she gets help. Also, don't compliment a woman's postpartum body. Actually, don't comment on women's bodies at all.

—Patty E.

happening and that you'll be okay. It's the same after having a baby. When we feel anxious and insecure about our bodies, we look for something to solve what we see as a problem. We are much more likely to be trusting of other people because they are selling us hope. And that's truly what dieting is: hope." Just say no—or rather, tap the button that says HIDE AD.

9. You might not want to have sex or even be touched.

It's not you, or your partner, or your relationship with one another. Your body is healing, your hormones are still in flux, and you are sleep-deprived in a way you've never been before. Be honest with your partner, let them know what you're feeling, and, if the problem persists beyond a few months, call your doctor.

10. This is for now, not forever.

When you are in the midst of all this, it will be hard to see beyond what you are feeling in the moment. It's important to remind yourself that this is temporary; it won't be like this forever. Say that to yourself multiple times a day, write it on a piece of paper, and hang it up somewhere you'll see it. I wrote myself a note that said, "This isn't forever," and it became a source of comfort for me whenever I saw it.

CHAPTER 9

Your Emotional Health

*Postpartum depression, anxiety, rage, and psychosis
are real and can't be ignored.*

I never expected the rage. True, I never expected the postpartum depression, either. But I thought, or maybe assumed, that depression was darkness. Lethargy. Slowly moving through a crippling fog. And it was. But I also had moments of rage.

I didn't know rage was a "thing," that it can come with PPD. I thought I was a violent, horrible human. I hid the episodes from everyone. I was so scared to tell anyone because I felt crazy. Truly. And I thought they'd judge me or take my baby away from me.

Never, in any moment of that near-blinding rage, did I forget my child and his safety. I say "near-blinding," because I still had just enough clear vision remaining to know that I needed to protect him. It was never him. It was me I wanted to hurt.

The pain inside me would usually send me to the floor, where I'd curl up in a ball and sob. But sometimes it was different; it became a ball inside me. And the ball would roll through my body, picking up more pain as it went until I needed to get it out, any way I could.

The ball would find its way to my arms and slide down to my fists. I'd scratch my skin, pull my hair. No relief. I'd make sure my baby was safely sleeping, far away. And then I'd punch the wall.

I felt no better. The ball was still there inside me.

My fist immediately throbbed, but upon inspection nothing was swelling. I'd hoped I would have at least fractured a finger, anything to cause a physical pain that would overshadow what I was feeling inside me. Or at least give me a benign enough reason to be in the hospital for a few days to rest, without having to worry about being locked away from my baby. I had lost my self-worth and the only value I saw in myself was being able to nurse this baby. So, at the very least, I had to be available to give him that.

I looked around for something to grab, to throw, to hit. To use as a vessel for what was inside me, this thing that I suddenly needed to release at any cost.

I saw a plastic cup. "San Francisco Giants, World Series Champions." I loved that cup.

I threw the cup against the wall and heard it crack. I cracked along with it, and my pain found an opening to leave my body at least for a moment.

For the time being, at least.

I really didn't know much about postpartum depression, either before or after my son was born. I remembered that

Brooke Shields wrote a book about it years ago and that Gwyneth Paltrow had mentioned it in some interviews, but other than that I just assumed it was varying degrees of sadness and depression. A social worker stopped by my hospital room on day two or three of my stay to talk about it, but by that point I was so tired of people coming in and out of my room that I sort of zoned out. I scanned the paperwork she handed me—only to make it look like I was reading for her sake—promised to be aware of any of the warning signs, and nodded in agreement with everything she was saying in hopes that she would leave and I could try to sleep.

There have been so many times that I've wished I could relive that interaction. I would have listened, asked questions about signs, symptoms, and treatment options. I would have asked if seeking help for PPD would result in my losing custody of my baby, as I'd later fear and would be a reason I stayed silent about my struggles.

I can't stress this enough: Postpartum hormones are no joke. Of course, we can and do sometimes joke about them because there really are moments when you feel like laughing and sobbing uncontrollably *and* simultaneously. And, many times, those feelings are just an overreaction to a situation brought on by sleep deprivation or hormone fluctuations and nothing more. But other times they can be a sign of something more serious.

EXPERT TIP

Not only are the symptoms of the baby blues and PPD similar to one another, they also mimic some of the symptoms of sleep deprivation. With the baby blues, there can be an inability to predict your emotions and how you react to things. Something that normally wouldn't bother you, such as spilling a glass of water, might cause you to break down and cry. With PPD there may be additional feelings of hopelessness and guilt. You could eat a piece of your favorite candy and find no pleasure in it, or even anything else for that matter. You might realize that there is nothing you are looking forward to. If you experience any of these feelings, don't wait even two weeks to see if they go away. Call your doctor immediately.

—Christine Sterling, MD

There are the baby blues, which is a common phrase we've all probably heard used to describe new mothers who feel sad or overwhelmed immediately after giving birth. The baby blues, while troubling in the moment, will pass quickly.

And then there's postpartum depression. And also, postpartum anxiety, rage, and psychosis. These are all incredibly serious and need to be addressed right away. In some cases, if left untreated, they can lead to self-harm or even death by suicide. Unfortunately, I know this firsthand because I was planning to end my life before finally seeking help for my PPD.

Please, if at any point postpartum you find that something doesn't feel right, call your doctor, doula, nurse, midwife, or a PPD hotline. Don't wait for that six-week checkup and don't wait for your partner, family, or friends to notice or agree with you that you need help. They might think you are exaggerating. They might be taking the lead from their mother, coworkers, or someone who isn't qualified to give advice yet telling them you are "probably" fine and just tired. Your mental health matters too much to leave to chance, and *you* know when something is amiss.

Let's start by looking at the *baby blues,* which are incredibly common. There is a strong chance—70 to 80 percent, to be specific—that a new mom will feel some level of sadness and anxiety after the birth of her baby. Though there are many commonalities between the baby blues and postpartum depression, they are not the same thing.

According to the CDC, women experiencing the baby blues may have feelings of worry, unhappiness, and fatigue. Yet when you look at PPD symptoms (which are outlined in the coming pages), they are very similar. Two key differences you need to remember are that feelings of PPD will be much more intense and last longer.

As an easy reminder, think of the baby blues as "two and two," meaning symptoms generally appear about two days after the birth of your baby and will resolve themselves in about two weeks. Postpartum depression continues beyond that.

Obviously, averages are not a guarantee, and some women experience feelings of the baby blues within hours of giving birth, and the two-week duration isn't set in stone. But to be on the safe side, if you find yourself still experiencing these feelings after two weeks, you need to seek help.

A friend of mine experienced the baby blues after the birth of her first child and PPD after welcoming her second. And while she wasn't trying to dismiss how serious maternal depression can be, she had a simple way of explaining the difference between the two. In her experience, the baby blues were like a mini-bout of depression and PPD was the baby blues that don't go away. In other words, unless your symptoms are severe from the start, you may need those two weeks to determine whether to seek help or not. But don't leave it to yourself alone to figure that out; speak with a professional.

When it comes to *PPD,* the statistics are different: One in eight women are affected, but that figure doesn't account for the number of women who have PPD and are never diagnosed. The CDC reports that 60 percent of women with symptoms never receive a clinical diagnosis.

PPD symptoms are similar to those of general depression, including a lasting sad or anxious mood; feeling hopeless, guilty, irritable, or restless; loss of energy; finding it hard to concentrate; appetite changes; oversleeping or not being able to fall asleep; and suicidal thoughts or attempts. (If you EVER feel like hurting yourself or your baby, call 911 immediately.) However, in addition to those, PPD symptoms may also include excessive crying, anger, withdrawing from those close to you and not feeling close with your baby, excess worrying, anxiety, thoughts of hurting yourself or your baby, and doubting your ability to care for your baby.

Postpartum rage is a symptom of PPD and can lead to pervasive feelings of anger, irritability, and, yes, rage.

Postpartum anxiety (PPA) may appear on its own or in addition to PPD. About 6 to 8 percent of new mothers will experience PPA, which generally manifests in the first six months after giving birth, though it can also happen when weaning or around the time your menstrual cycle returns. Symptoms are excessive worry, racing thoughts, panic attacks, being convinced that something bad will happen, interruptions to sleep and eating, and an inability to sit still. PPA may also be accompanied by physical symptoms, like nausea and dizziness.

Postpartum psychosis is very rare and very serious. For every thousand births only one to three women are diagnosed. The onset can be almost immediate, and the range is twenty-four hours to three weeks after giving birth. Symptoms include mood fluctuations; auditory hallucinations; and thoughts of suicide, homicide, or infanticide. Postpartum psychosis must be addressed immediately.

It's important to know that all of these conditions can be treated with medication, therapy, or a combination of both. There are also support groups where you can connect with other moms in your situation (see the resources list on page 310 for more details).

Real Mom Story

The minute my twins were born I knew something wasn't right. One of my daughters had terrible colic and would scream for hours each day, leaving me convinced she was a demon. I refused to be left alone with her but didn't tell anyone that it was because I was afraid of her and what I thought she was capable of doing. I was convinced she knew that she had a power over me and others and started to think I needed to do something about it. When I finally told my husband and family, they said they'd never heard of anything like this, and I was exaggerating. I went straight to my doctor and was diagnosed with postpartum psychosis. I took medication and went to therapy but now I'm consumed with guilt. My doctor told me that I shouldn't feel guilty, because guilt signifies choice, and I had no choice in how I felt. It's sad, but I got more support from strangers in mom groups on Facebook than I did from my family. My husband and I are in therapy together and trying to overcome how this experience almost ended our marriage. I wish I'd known about postpartum psychosis and that it's real. Motherhood can be so hard the first few years, and even after that it's never the perfect image you see on social media. Some of us don't always bond with our babies immediately.

—Shannon M.

For me, PPD started slowly. It wasn't immediate, and even when it did begin it wasn't as if I were curled up in a ball, sobbing uncontrollably—although that did come later—which was what I expected it would be like. Maybe it's because I didn't know much about it, but I assumed it was this all-encompassing emotional paralysis that would accompany me when I came home from the hospital.

That wasn't the case.

I was a first-time mom recovering from a C-section. I was sad, exhausted, hormonal, and scared, which I assumed was par for the course with a newborn. Yet as the weeks progressed, I watched my incision heal, but emotionally I still felt the same.

I didn't feel connected to my son. Of course I loved him. Didn't I? He was my child. He was beautiful and soft, he curled into my chest, and I felt a fierce need to protect him. But he was also feeding off my body every 120 minutes and had less personality than a sea urchin. I mean, of course I *loved* him. I just didn't know him yet. At least that's what I told myself.

I quickly fell further into indifference. I knew my role of feeding and nurturing was important, but other than that, I felt I could slip out the door and no one would notice or care that I'd left. My son and I weren't bonding, I was terrible at swaddling, and he seemed to prefer being held by anyone but me. In hindsight, I know that wasn't the case, but my mind told me otherwise in the moment.

Besides my boobs, I was useless to this child.

I can't say I was happy. I loved my son, I'd say to myself repeatedly in an effort to make it true, but I felt like I'd been imprisoned in this new life and routine. *But,* I'd tell myself, *women have been doing this for centuries. This must be normal, and my resistance must be because I'm not a good mother.*

I begged my husband to pack up the baby and depart for his mother's house. It made the most sense to me; I clearly couldn't be a mother and I felt what I was sure was his silent judgment burning a hole in my heart.

He told me I was being ridiculous. "You're tired," he explained. *No,* I thought. *I'm a bad person.*

When it was time for my six-week checkup, I was down, but things hadn't quite manifested to the point of concern, so I carried on. That's the thing with PPD; it creeps up slowly. You have bad moments and good, a bad week and a good day. The good days make it easy for you to convince yourself that you're fine and maybe even overreacting.

Unfortunately, the good days never lasted and the bad would return. Back and forth until you're entirely submerged within the black cloud of your brain and it feels too late to go back.

I had no personal frame of reference and didn't know what was normal. No one I knew ever had PPD or, if they did, they never spoke about it. I was convinced that I was the only woman to ever struggle with motherhood and that I was simply a bad mom. I thought my son deserved better, that my family would be better off without me, and the only thing I could do was breastfeed.

At first, I didn't ask for help because I didn't realize what was happening to me. I didn't pay attention in the hospital when I had the chance to learn about PPD. After about another month of this, I went online and looked at PPD symptoms, but I couldn't decipher if that's what it was or if I just needed sleep. Part of me also didn't want to know because I was afraid that if I told anyone, a doctor would confirm what I believed: that it wasn't PPD, that I shouldn't have become a mom.

With a newborn, sleep is elusive. Yet when I actually had the opportunity to rest I couldn't. Insomnia took over. I began cleaning baseboards with Q-tips at 3 a.m.—anything to keep busy. That was another sign of PPD that I didn't recognize, which is not being able to sleep when you finally have the chance.

My husband tried to help me, but he had no idea what was happening. He tried to talk to me about it, but every conversation ended with me blaming myself, damning myself for sticking this beautiful soul with me as his mother.

My parents were becoming increasingly worried with each visit. My mom, as a retired nurse, knew I wasn't doing well and encouraged me to seek help, but I refused each time, reassuring her that I was just tired.

What none of them knew was that I'd also been secretly experiencing those moments of rage. I knew it wasn't normal behavior, which made me even more reluctant to be honest about what I was feeling and experiencing. I was so scared to share and ask for help because I felt crazy. Truly. And I was convinced that if anyone found out, I would be held in a hospital against my will, or my son would be taken away from us.

Over the next two months, I vacillated between wanting to run away or take my own life. I had plans for both. To run away I would simply hightail it to the park down the street and go to sleep. A bench or the ground would do. And when the police showed up to question the "crazy lady," I'd pretend I was a mute. Then, I reasoned, they'd take me to jail, where I could sleep even more. In hindsight this plan sounds absolutely delusional, but I thought it was flawless.

When I relayed this part of my story to Dr. Sterling, she immediately recognized it as sleep deprivation. "When you are sleep-deprived, your brain is desperately trying to get you to sleep. It will tell you crazy things to get you to sleep in an effort to protect itself."

The more concerning plan was the one to take my own life. I need to run an errand, I'd say. Then I'd set out in my car and find a wall to drive into. All I could hear in my head was how healthy all the breastfeeding was for my son—the only thing I seemed to be good for. So, I would keep nursing him to help him get started in life, then I would enact my plan. I decided six months would be good, and mentally marked the day on a calendar in my mind.

I existed in survival mode, though I was barely doing that.

I held on as best as I could until the day I let go, which came after about four months. My son was crying, as babies do. But I couldn't handle it. The wails caused a physical reaction in my body that was like nothing I'd ever felt. I wanted to rip my skin off and pull out my hair. I tried to soothe him to no avail. I placed him down in his bassinet and fell to the ground sobbing.

"I give up, I give up," I screamed. To everyone and no one. "Please," I begged of the universe. "Help me be a mother. I don't know how."

My son and I cried in unison for about a minute, though it felt like much longer. I then crawled on my hands and knees to where I'd dropped my cell phone earlier and called my husband at work.

"Please come home now," I said in a calm voice that felt foreign after my outburst. "I need help."

He came home and I drove straight to my ob-gyn's office. I walked in and, as soon as the office manager saw me, she came wordlessly toward me and enveloped me in a hug. I sobbed, and she held me in that moment when I was unable to stand on my own.

She escorted me to an exam room and sat me down. My favorite nurse, the one who'd seen me through all those exams and twice-weekly non-stress tests during my pregnancy, soon appeared bearing a plate of pumpkin bread. "Eat," she instructed. And I did. I was suddenly ravenous, the dam broke, and I was able to accept help in every form.

I was there for a while; my doctor assessed me and decided I wasn't going to harm myself or anyone else. I answered questions, spoke honestly about the previous few months. I heard the words *postpartum depression*. Yes, I want to try medication, I answered when asked.

I was prescribed the antidepressant medication Zoloft, and we created a plan. I talked with my husband, my parents stopped their lives to come and stay with us so I wouldn't be alone during the day. I was going to get better, I was told, but I couldn't do it alone. And I didn't need to try.

While that day was the beginning of my healing, it was far from the beginning of the end, I'd soon learn. The medication helped tremendously. Within two weeks I saw the old me in the mirror. It was still a bit hazy, like the steam from a shower was clouding my view, but she was there. I didn't realize how much I'd missed her until that moment.

I began seeing a therapist and shared my story with family, friends, and even strangers on social media. I was shocked at how many women had gone through the same thing I had. It made me feel less alone, but I was also angry. Why wasn't this talked about more? If I had known my feelings weren't uncommon, would I have sought help sooner? I thought of all the time I lost with my son. Months of going through the motions, willing time to pass. Not being able to enjoy him.

The remainder of that first year was full of ups and downs. I felt better, overall. I smiled real and true smiles, loved my child and was fully present in each moment of his life. All the aspects of motherhood that eluded me were now part of my daily life and I was thankful.

I had setbacks. But I knew the signs, what to look for, and, most important, what to do. I used my voice and was honest about my feelings. My medication was changed a few times. Increased, actually, but I never cared. I was always happy that something existed that helped me ignore the lies my mind was telling me. I knew, at last, I was a good mother.

It's been nearly six years since my PPD diagnosis, and I still take medication and see a therapist. I've learned that my mental health wasn't a sickness that could be fixed by one or two things; it's an ongoing journey that I proactively manage.

I remember speaking with my doctor about a year after I began taking the Zoloft, and I marveled at what a marked difference it made in every aspect of my life. I was so overwhelmed by how it had the ability to make me want to get out of bed each day and not only live life, but also enjoy it.

Real Mom Story

I suffered from undiagnosed PPD after my son was born. One thing I really wished someone had told me was that the screenings are terrible, they are very easy to manipulate if you don't want your PPD recognized, and very easy to slip through the cracks if you do. I had a feeling I had PPD, but part of that was me not believing I deserved help. I remember reading the questionnaire they had given me that actually said, "If you think your baby is or has been sent by a god or devil, you may have serious postpartum mental complications." I thought about how I couldn't sleep or stop crying, but I certainly didn't think that my son was Satan, either. I decided that just meant that I didn't have it and needed to stay quiet. The hospital staff and your doctor can help you, but only if you let them. You have to be honest, even if you think you're not worthy of help and support. And someone needs to look into making better screening tests!

—Jamie R.

"I hope that helps you finally give yourself some grace," she said.

"Grace?" I asked. "For what?"

"Because you've always blamed yourself for your PPD," she began. "As much as you're told that it's not your fault, that you didn't cause it, you still seem to think you could have prevented it. Does this show you now that it was chemical? It was your brain, not you."

And that, my friends, was the biggest takeaway from my journey through postpartum depression, one that took far too long to realize and about another four years to accept. This was beyond anything I could control or prevent and was going to happen to me regardless of anything I did to prepare for or try to prevent it (outside of taking medication once diagnosed).

But, boy, did I waste a lot of time and tears while coming to that realization.

I can now look back and recognize that I did nothing wrong, that my PPD wasn't my fault or something I could have prevented. I just wish I'd known more about it, was aware of how it could manifest, and that I shouldn't feel that way. And that is what I hope to share with others, so no one else has to endure what I did.

To make it easy for moms who don't know where to start, I've included an extensive list of resources right here in this book (see page 310) because sometimes googling what you need is too much. At least that's how I've felt at times. The smallest of tasks can feel absolutely insurmountable when paired with depression. But there is help, and I can guide you to it. I promise, I won't let you navigate this alone.

It's not always easy to begin your journey to healing. Often, women who do speak out about feeling less than blissful after the birth of their baby are told that "It's just the baby blues." Yes, that actually may be the case for many, and making them aware that it is a common ailment that will soon pass can be helpful. However, talking about mental health can make people uncomfortable and, in an effort to avoid discussing it, they will often tell someone that "It's just the baby blues" whether or not they know anything about it. I've spoken to moms who were many months into their depressive postpartum feelings, yet when they found the courage to talk about it, all they heard was this sweeping generalization.

This is yet another reason it is so important for us to advocate for our mental health always, and especially postpartum. Things are improving as more people publicly share their stories, but for the most part, society still isn't all that accepting and understanding of mental health disorders. There is a strong chance someone will dismiss you. Or give you bad advice. That's why I'm asking you to please, if you take anything away from this book, be aware of your mental health and how you're feeling after your baby is born. If you don't feel normal, if it lasts longer than two weeks, or even if you're just not yourself yet you can't put your finger on why, seek help.

EXPERT TIP

Intrusive thoughts about your baby being harmed are common with postpartum mood disorders; what you need to look at is how you feel when you're having them. Generally, intrusive thoughts are very upsetting. With PPD, they can lead to guilt and send you into a shame spiral. If you have PPA, you can't seem to let these thoughts and worries go. But with postpartum psychosis, those thoughts aren't going to cause worry or make someone upset. Those thoughts aren't fears; they're reality.

—Christine Sterling, MD

A wonderful resource that I personally used to find free and local help for my PPD is Postpartum Support International (PSI), which is also listed in the resources section at the end of this book. PSI offers a wealth of resources for moms. You can call the helpline (in English and Spanish), join an online support group, read through the group's abundant resource documents, and find a provider or connect with a local support coordinator. I reached out to my local coordinator (someone assigned to your city or county). This person can direct you to all available help in your area. Mine helped me find a therapist who specialized in treating women with PPD, and it was life changing.

You might come into contact with people who will never understand or accept mental health disorders as "real." No matter what you are going through, they will excuse it away. I struggled with this part, especially. I didn't have a fever, I wasn't coughing, and I didn't look sick. So, they'd reason, I was actually just fine. There were times when I wished my condition would make me bleed—anything visible to prove to these naysayers that, yes, just because they didn't see it with their own eyes, I was indeed in a bad place. It took me a long time to realize that I was never going to convince these people that I was just as sick as anyone else and needed help. I worked to get to a place where I could ignore those opinions and focus on the opinions of those in my support system, who did believe me. It's not your responsibility to change people's perception of mental health. All you need to do is get healthy.

While I would prefer that no mom ever had to deal with PPD again, I know that's not possible. If I can't prevent it, at least I want to prepare you for it. Knowledge is power when it comes to your mental health, and it's important to be able to recognize any signs or symptoms of PPD. Unfortunately, there might be some people in your life who are just miserable humans and won't support you. Please don't let them deter you from getting help and being happy, which you—and your baby— absolutely deserve. Feel free to send them my way if they won't leave you alone. I'll handle them while you read up on the list of key takeaways.

1. Baby blues are real.

Yes, the baby blues are temporary, but that doesn't mean this condition isn't real. Be kind to yourself in the first weeks and be aware of your mental health. A lot of what you're feeling is beyond your control, so please go easy on yourself. And if you do experience feelings of depression, anxiety, or anything that doesn't feel like "you," keep track of when it began. If it lasts longer than two weeks, please seek help.

2. PPD is also real.

This breaks my heart to say, but I've spoken with countless women whose partners and family have said that PPD isn't real. Don't let anyone ever tell you that. It is a real medical condition that needs treatment. You don't have to be alone in this; there is a wide network of help and support. And, regardless of what anyone may tell you, I believe you.

3. It doesn't hurt to seek help.

As mothers, we tend to put our own needs last. I often dismiss things because I think there isn't time, it's not that important, and my to-do list feels insurmountable at best on a good day. Let me tell you what I learned the hard way: Everything falls apart when you aren't well. If you think something is off, see your doctor. If you don't have insurance or can't afford an extra visit, contact PSI (see page 313) to be connected to free resources in your area.

4. You're not a bad mom and this isn't your fault.

Don't listen to the lies your brain is telling you. PPD doesn't dis-
criminate. Anyone who gives birth is at risk. You didn't cause this,
you don't deserve it, and you're a wonderful mother.

5. It's hard to talk about mental health.

There is an unfortunate stigma surrounding mental health. Some
people don't believe it's a real thing, others think we somehow
bring it upon ourselves and can make the feelings stop at will,
and then there are those who won't even entertain a discussion.
I wish I could tell you that your journey will be easy, but that's
not the case. You might have to use all your resources to find
the strength to ask for help, and then encounter one of those
naysayers. Guess what? They're wrong. Keep fighting for your
health. You will find others who believe you and have been
there themselves.

**6. You will be surprised at how many women you know
who've had or have PPD.**

It's like this secret club that no one wants to be in, but once
others know you're a member you'll quickly realize that you're
not alone. Almost daily, I connect with other women on social
media who are fellow PPD warriors. They tell me about the
self-doubt and loneliness they faced early on, and the challenges
that may have delayed their treatment. It's comforting to know

that countless other women have weathered the storms, received care, and made it to the other side. You are not alone.

7. Don't be afraid of medication.

The stigma surrounding mental health also extends to medication used in treatment. This absolutely infuriates me. If someone is a diabetic, would we tell them to forgo daily insulin in favor of exercise, sunshine, and therapy? Of course not. Why, then, do people frown upon medication? Each of us is unique, and our treatment will be, too. Don't be dissuaded because you've heard of someone else having a bad experience with medication. You will have a plan tailored to you and your needs. It can and probably will be tweaked from time to time in an effort to increase efficacy, and it doesn't have to be permanent. Sometimes, all you may need is a temporary solution to pull you out of depression and then you can move along to other treatments, if needed.

8. You have options for treatment.

There is a misconception that mental health disorders can only be treated with medication. While that was the case for me, I've met others whose treatment didn't involve medication. There are myriad ways to treat PPD, and it's common to combine several, including therapy, support groups, exercise, meditation, diet, and involvement in your community.

9. Not everyone will understand.

There are people who will never accept that PPD and mental illness are a real or serious thing. The good news is that it's not your job to educate them. I've written about my PPD journey countless times, and I still have people in my life who don't think it was "that" bad. One even asked me if I'd gotten "that thing" I thought was a problem out of my system. It used to hurt my feelings, but I've realized their opinions have no place in my healing.

10. Your baby deserves a happy mom.

If you still don't believe that your mental health is important, think of your baby. They deserve the best version of you, and that might include your getting help for your PPD. If not for yourself, do it for them.

CHAPTER 10
Handling Unsolicited Advice

Your mother-in-law is not a pediatrician.

"If your baby ever has trouble sleeping, just give them a bath in boiled lettuce water and it will knock them right out! But don't forget to take the lettuce out before you put the baby in."

Just before I let out a polite laugh, I realized my grandma's neighbor was being serious. I'd just announced my pregnancy to her, a woman I'd known my entire life, and she cried tears of joy while giving me a surprisingly strong hug for a ninety-four-year-old woman.

And then she started rattling off every baby tip she could think of, including the lettuce bath. It was sweet and made me miss my own grandmother, who'd died during the first trimester of my pregnancy, all the more. Even though I didn't ask for advice, and a lot of what she said sounded like something I'd never try, I knew it was coming from a place of love.

I think it's safe to say that, for the most part, while this advice is well-intentioned, there will always be people who speak up for no good reason. I'm not saying that a person actually wakes up one morning and thinks, *What is the most damaging thing I can tell someone to do and pretend it's good advice?* That type of behavior is

205

on par with a sociopath. So, let's assume the people we're referring to aren't *clinically* cruel, just occasionally obnoxious.

With these individuals, unsolicited advice is given solely to imply that you don't know what you're doing, or that the way you parent is wrong. Nothing can come from that, other than making you feel awful, and, unfortunately, that is the exact outcome these people are aiming for.

The harsh reality is that some people you know are petty and jealous, or maybe even downright mean. And that won't change just because you have a baby.

Mean people aside, even when given with the best of intentions from the most caring of people, these nuggets of advice that you never asked for can be aggravating. Receiving unsolicited advice is one of the most universal frustrations among moms I've spoken with.

This sounds a little selfish, right? If people are only trying to help, what's so bad about that? Well, it's not really that cutand-dried. And a lot of it has to do with who is offering the unsolicited advice, how and when they offer it, and if they're advising—or telling—you to try something.

Your baby will be fine, whether you listen to the advice or not. You are surrounded by well-intentioned family and friends who love your baby very much. But you need to develop a strategy for dealing with all their unsolicited advice, before it drives you crazy.

Your mother, mother-in-law, grandmother, aunt, anyone who comes at you with their seasoned advice, gave birth decades ago and much has changed since then. We have more advanced tools and practices. We've learned, and things have evolved.

Beyond that, every baby is different. What may work wonders for some babies (and parents) could be the prelude for a colossal meltdown for others. Which means that advice—either requested or not—should be received and then filtered, based on you and your baby's needs and traits.

Don't let anyone tell you how to care for your baby. And not just strangers on the internet. This also includes those closest to you. I was lucky because my mom was quick to remind me that she didn't always know what she was talking about in terms of babies. "It's been a while since you and your sister were babies," she said, and pointed out all the differences between then and now, from how we put babies down to sleep (always on the back) to no longer using crib bumpers or blankets. Times change. Yes, babies are the same, but the way in which we care for them evolves. Don't let anyone tell you otherwise.

People want to help. They also love to be right and all-knowing. Many will blatantly tell you when they think you're wrong and how to do everything.

And it's not just unsolicited opinions. You also may find yourself on the receiving end of excess toys and clothes and baby gear you didn't ask for or even want. Remember that you are your child's mother, and you have final say on what lives in your home. You can stay true to yourself and still respect those with good intentions.

"Unsolicited advice is rooted in people feeling good when they think they know something," says Leslie Wasserman, LCSW. "It's often well-intentioned, and there can be some desire to actually be helpful. But it can become a problem if they don't take the time to make sure the advice is wanted."

EXPERT TIP

When people in your life are offering unsolicited advice, it's important to remember that you're not speaking with an expert. If what someone is suggesting you do feels out of alignment to you, then don't do it. And if they keep pushing until you feel like you need to justify your decision, use your doctor as an excuse. I tell patients they can always throw me under the bus, so to speak, and just blame me.

—Christine Sterling, MD

Before we map out methods for dealing with unsolicited advice, let's look at why it can feel so grating. Understanding the reasons we may be triggered by what seems like nothing more than a helpful suggestion can ultimately help us control our reactions and, hopefully, save us from even more unnecessary emotional stress. Instead of being irritated and possibly pissed off, remind yourself that it's not worth getting upset over because anything this particular person says will bother you, or that you're not mad about the advice per se, just that you've heard it so many times that it feels like nagging.

After speaking with many mothers, I've compiled a list of the top reasons why unsolicited advice leaves so many of us wanting to scream into a pillow.

It can feel like criticism. If someone isn't asking for advice, it might be because they don't think they need any. In that case, dropping a bomb full of uninvited suggestions can make a person feel like they're being told that what they're doing is wrong, or needs improvement.

It can feel like an effort to control the situation. This reaction often tends to result when close family and friends are involved, and just how insistent they become that you follow their suggestions. After a while, you begin to wonder if this is really about diaper rash cream or someone who isn't ready to step back and let you—the parent—take the lead.

It can feel condescending. This can have a lot to do with tone and delivery but, in general, spouting off ways someone should do something—without them asking for suggestions—can also make a person feel like they're being talked down to.

It can feel like nagging. Advice in any form is one thing; repeatedly suggesting it starts to feel like nagging. Especially when you didn't want the advice to begin with.

Some people want to figure things out themselves. If there was something I didn't know, or had a question about, I would ask someone I trusted. My husband, on the other hand, really wanted to figure some things out himself. Sort of an "on-the-job training," so to speak. When someone stepped in uninvited, and just told him what to do, he felt like an opportunity was stolen from him.

It can depend on the person giving it. I don't want to throw all mothers-in-law under the bus because many are quite lovely, but a lot of women cite them as one of the biggest sources of unsolicited advice. And, if the relationship isn't great to begin with, the advice will feel grating simply because of the person sharing it with you.

It can pit the parents against one another. Whether it's something specific or just unsolicited advice in general, if one person is in favor of trying it and the other is not, it can be a catalyst for disagreements and arguments.

It can be wrong. Remember: People don't have to fact-check their advice before they dole it out. Just because they had a baby or have seen a baby, that doesn't mean they know everything about babies. And they certainly don't know your baby best—you do.

It can spark feelings of anxiety, insecurity, or depression. Some people take feedback better than others; they simply let it roll off their backs. Others may take it to heart, and being told what they should do (or do differently) comes across as criticism and affects their mental health.

It can cause resentment. If someone is constantly giving you unsolicited advice, it's unlikely you'll begin to look at them as your preferred go-to baby expert. You'll probably become annoyed or, worse, you'll just end up resenting all their forced "help."

It's been said that if you're looking for unsolicited advice, then you should get pregnant. And if you can't get enough by doing that, have a baby.

I can fully endorse those statements as truth because I lived these scenarios myself.

My husband and I faced two big challenges upon becoming parents: my son's refusal to sleep and my worsening PPD. While I was trying to do everything I could, from asking friends for advice to reading books and talking to other new moms online, my husband talked about it with what felt like every single person he knew. And, once he opened that door of discussion, the random suggestions came flying.

My husband was lost, of course he was. I see that now. Without a guidebook or any clue as to what was happening, he started reaching out for help. To friends, family, and coworkers . . . hell, he was so desperate he probably asked for advice at the grocery store. And while I can't blame him for trying, this "help" he received from well-meaning individuals contributed greatly to my mental downfall because it left me feeling many of the things listed above. I felt like I was being criticized, that everyone assumed I was a bad mother. My husband and I began to disagree on how to handle things, and it all fed my growing depression.

It slowly trickled in at first, mostly observations: "You're tired." "All newborns are terrible sleepers." "It will get better with time." All of this I easily filed into the "duh" category; while I may have been falling into a hole of depression, even I knew all that to be true.

Yet when things didn't improve for me or for my son's sleep, my husband started coming home with advice. For my PPD, I heard these gems: "You need to exercise." "Other people have it worse. You need to realize that you're not really struggling." "Sunshine will help—just spend more time outside." "Just try to be happy." All these felt impossible to me. Getting dressed took the bulk of my physical strength: How was I going to go to the gym and further exert myself? I'd take my son outside and turn my head upward toward the sun, hoping that somehow its rays would magically cure me and my will to live would be restored. But it never happened, and I just became more convinced that everyone was better at motherhood than I was.

The sleep "help" was all over the place. We received a lot of product suggestions, which I actually appreciated because it allowed me to look into an option on my own time and sometimes made me aware of things I never knew existed. But it was the people who essentially said we needed to parent in a different way who made me feel like I was a failure. We kept his bedroom too hot or too cold, we were putting him to sleep hungry, we hadn't properly soothed and relaxed him before bed, and—my favorite of all—I was breastfeeding him too much, thus he had become spoiled and didn't want to sleep alone.

We didn't see much progress, which my husband didn't hide from anyone. So, after that, people tried to rationalize my misery to my husband as he struggled to make sense of things, fearing it would become our new normal. He came home one day hopeful, thinking he and whomever he'd spoken with this time had found the root cause of my problem. "I think I know what's happening," he began. "You expected motherhood to be easy. And it's not. So you're just unprepared and in shock. Once you adjust to how hard motherhood truly is, you'll be better at dealing with it. Oh, and we need to let the baby cry it out and fall asleep."

Was he serious? I scanned his eyes, waiting for the joke. But all I saw was hope. He thought he'd finally stumbled upon the answer to what was happening to me. And not only that, but the cure to our problems was actually quite simple.

That's when I put my foot down. I told him that I didn't want to hear any more opinions from people, especially when given secondhand. If someone thought I was unprepared to be a mom, let them say it to me. He could tell me about books, products, websites, or articles. But there would be no more of this, "I was talking to so-and-so, and she said that what you need to do is . . ."

I also reminded him that our pediatrician told us in no uncertain terms that our son was months away from sleep training, let alone "crying it out," and we would not be letting him scream his tiny head off, alone in his crib. And I didn't care if it did work for the ex-sister-in-law of a guy he worked with. We would be listening to the experts in our lives, not the unknown relatives of people we hardly knew.

In our society, or perhaps in human nature, we have an overwhelming urge to give our opinions, advice, and flat-out tell people what to do. Even when we have no business doing so. Sure, sunshine, exercise, hugs, and puppies can help sometimes, but other situations call for more help. It's okay to just listen to someone talk about their problems without giving advice. If they ask directly, you can always say, "Gee, that doesn't sound like anything I'm familiar with. Perhaps you should see a doctor or expert." It's not like you'll be punished for deflecting the question or receive a gold star if you do answer.

I'm often asked what I wish we had done with all the unsolicited advice we received. I wish that my husband hadn't listened to what people were saying, or at least that he hadn't told me every single word of it. I wish he'd recognized this wasn't right and taken me to get help—though now I see that he was being told this wasn't a "real problem," I might have just "been acting dramatic because the baby was getting all the attention" (actual quote from someone he spoke with).

I also wish people could have stayed in their lane. Yes, I know you wanted to help. But don't you see that this was above your pay grade and you weren't qualified to advise on this topic? If one person had refrained from trying to fix our situation, to justify it as "only" exhaustion, and instead pushed us to see my doctor, I could have started my healing so much sooner. Maybe I would have gotten help before I started planning how I'd take my own life. And I'd never have to live with those memories or carry this guilt over all the time with my son lost to the fog of my illness. The guilt will be with me for a long time, if not always.

If you ever find yourself being asked what to do in a situation that seems foreign to you, just remember that it's okay not to know. You can, you *should,* be honest and help direct that person to an expert. Whether it's postpartum depression, cancer, or a faulty car transmission, there are qualified individuals available to help. And maybe all you need to do is be the one to point that out.

Once my husband and I reached an understanding on unsolicited advice—which was to ignore it or keep it to yourself—things began to improve. I was able to relax because I no longer felt a burst of anxiety every time we spoke. I knew there wouldn't be any "Someone said you should do this"-type suggestions. In turn, I wasn't irritated with him, and our conversations were much more pleasant without that underlying tension between us. Instead of him sharing unsolicited advice and me immediately shutting down as a result, we worked together to find solutions.

And sure, my son's sleep didn't get much better until he was old enough for a sleep coach, and my PPD wasn't diagnosed until I reached my breaking point and spoke to my doctor, but I don't believe either of those things would have been "fixed" with all the unsolicited advice we received. I do think I may have talked with my doctor sooner had it not been for all the suggestions that I was simply ill-prepared to be a mom. Perhaps we would have realized earlier on that my struggles weren't normal.

Real Mom Story

My girlfriend's mother is the most hands-on, magical mom and grandma I've ever seen. We call her "Nanny Poppins."

When our daughter was born, she was perfect. But she screamed nonstop if she wasn't being held, and my girlfriend and I took shifts during the night so that she'd never be put down.

Nanny told us we were being ridiculous.

She told us that it's not only fine for a baby to scream, it's beneficial because the crying would strengthen her lungs. If we let her cry now, she'd be less susceptible to respiratory infections in the future.

We followed her instructions. But it was painful to hear my daughter cry like that. Eventually, my girlfriend picked her up and said she didn't care if her lungs were strong. I argued that her mom knew what she was talking about and we should try it again. That only resulted in all three of us crying.

The next day, we happened to have a pediatrician appointment, and we mentioned our daughter's soon-to-be-healthy lungs. Our pediatrician gave us a sympathetic smile and told us that's an old wives' tale. "Think about it," she said. "Our lungs are not a muscle, there's nothing to stretch."

After that experience, Nanny didn't stop giving us unsolicited advice; I just stopped listening.

—Beth A.

While there is no way to completely escape unsolicited advice, there are things you and your partner can both do to help soften the impact of this well-intentioned but often unbearable aspect of parenting.

1. Make a plan before your baby arrives.

My husband and I never thought twice about unsolicited advice during my pregnancy, so we were wholly unprepared when it became an issue after our son was born. If you and your partner even have one conversation about it, you'll be ahead of the game. Discuss how you feel about unsolicited advice in general and how you'd like to handle it. Also, be sure to talk about it again after your baby is born, because that's when you'll be inundated with it.

2. Have an honest conversation with those closest to you.

Personally, I'm not one for confrontation, but I can be up-front with my immediate family and closest friends. If you have a strong opinion about being offered "gentle suggestions," let them know one way or the other. Maybe you know that you absolutely don't want to hear anything without being asked, or perhaps you want their advice and opinions. Personally, I try my hardest to keep my mouth closed when someone has a baby, but a friend of mine specifically told me that she wanted me to know that I could offer her any advice, whether unsolicited or not. And without hearing that, I probably never would have.

3. If you can, let it go.

In an ideal world, if someone decided they absolutely needed to tell us how we could better push our baby's stroller, we would nod along and thank them for sharing. Then, we'd either take the advice or forget it. Some people are better at this than others. I was able to do this in some situations, like that lettuce bath, but with certain people I couldn't get past it, regardless of what they said. Try to overlook at least some of it.

4. Create an exit plan.

If you know for a fact that you receive unsolicited advice about as well as fish can swim out of water, plan things in advance that you can say to end or change the conversation, especially if you struggle to come up with ideas on the spot. "Thank you for that idea, but I'm running late for a doctor's appointment" or "That's interesting, but can you tell me what happened with your neighbor who you think stole your Amazon package?" Turning the focus back to them is a great way to change the course of the conversation.

5. Be direct and honest.

As I said, this isn't my specialty. I will tell someone the most complicated story in an effort to avoid confrontation and possibly keep from hurting their feelings. I am in awe of those who can come out and say exactly what they think. If that is you, use that moxie to meet the situation head-on. A polite response that makes your feelings known in no uncertain terms might sound like this: "Thank you for the suggestions. I value your experience, but I think I want to try things my own way. Would you be open to me calling you to ask for advice when I need it?"

6. Take a vow of silence at home.

In addition to how you feel about unsolicited advice, you need to factor in your partner's opinions, too. One of you may have no problem with it, while the other wants nothing to do with it. In that situation, you might want to consider putting a moratorium on it, meaning don't talk about it and especially don't share with your partner anything someone may have advised you to do or try.

7. Write it down for your partner.

Sometimes the problem with unsolicited advice is the timing. I know that, if I'm especially tired or stressed, I'm not as open to hearing uninvited opinions. But when I'm rested and clearheaded, I'm much better at managing my emotions. My husband actually had the idea that, instead of just telling me everything and anything people told him, he would write it down. We tried this and it was actually a big help. He kept a notebook that I would read on my own time, instead of hearing, "My cousin said you should do this . . ." in the midst of a baby meltdown.

8. Keep it anonymous.

In many instances, the only thing we don't like about unsolicited advice is the person giving it. If you or your partner know that certain people can trigger you, consider making a list of people you don't want to hear from. Then, if someone on your partner's list starts telling you how to raise your baby, be sure you don't run home and tell them all about it. Or at least, don't tell them who said it.

9. Ask permission.

My biggest problem with all this unsolicited advice was that it made me feel like I was receiving it because I was failing as a mom. Many moms have said that they would be much more open to hearing secondhand advice from their partner if they just asked first, instead of unloading without warning. A lot of us handle this better when we're prepared and in the right headspace. For example, instead of saying, "Someone told me we should do . . . ," try "I heard an interesting idea. Do you want to hear about it?" Or, if it's from a trigger person, don't mention the source. Even when asking permission, be sure to keep it anonymous if the advice comes from one of your partner's identified triggers.

Real Mom Story

According to my mom, babies only hiccup because they're cold. My daughter was a frequent hiccuper and all we heard was that we weren't keeping her warm enough—despite my constant insistence to my mom that her ideas were outdated and wrong.

She would blast the heater, dress the baby in multiple layers, and a few times we stopped her from covering our baby with blankets while she slept (which is against safe sleep practices). There were even times I'd see her on the baby monitor, sneaking in after I put my daughter down for a nap and covering her with a blanket!

No matter what we said, she kept at it. Until one day when my frustration with my mom collided with my hormones and sleep deprivation and sent me over the edge and I lost it.

She yelled back and we both cried. But after we both calmed down, we talked.

If I could do it over again, I would have spent less time fighting with her and trying to win what felt like an argument and instead setting clear boundaries from the start. I wish I'd told her that while we loved her and appreciated her help, if she was going to insist upon doing things in a way that we disagreed with, then she'd have to leave.

—Karen C.

10. Stay aligned with each other.

Advice, whether invited or not, can cause problems when one parent wants to try it and the other doesn't. It's important to be on the same page to avoid resentment. This is another great conversation to have before your baby is born. What will you do if one of you wants to try something and the other doesn't? Do you each get a veto? Maybe you both agree to a timeline, such as "We'll try this if the problem still persists in a week." It may seem like overkill, but you'll be happy you put boundaries in place *before* you find yourselves awake at 3 a.m. with a baby who refuses to sleep. If my husband and I had thought to do that before our son was born, we likely never would have had an argument about me insisting he go to the grocery store in the middle of the night to buy a head of iceberg lettuce. You see, I had become so desperate to get our son to sleep that I was ready to try that infamous lettuce bath my grandma's neighbor told me about. Unfortunately—or maybe I should say fortunately—I'll never know because my husband won that argument.

CHAPTER 11

Navigating Friendships

When your bestie doesn't like babies.

I was scrolling through Instagram in the middle of the night, while I was awake and breastfeeding my son, when I came across a picture of two of my close friends smiling while they sat in what looked like a hotel lobby. The caption said, "Annual girls' trip." On any other occasion I'd be happy to see their faces, but this time my stomach dropped, and tears welled up in my eyes. I felt hurt and left out. That annual girls' trip they were on was one that I had been a part of for the past six years. I had assumed that because my son was two and a half months old at the time we usually went that we'd all skip it that year, but I was wrong. I was the only one who was skipping anything, only I didn't know it.

I tried to think of what I'd done wrong to make one or both of them upset with me. The only thing I could come up with was some unreturned text messages. But it wasn't a lot of messages, and besides, I'd just had a baby. And they were mothers themselves, although their kids were in high school at that point.

I gave in to the tears while I wrote and deleted a slew of different yet equally snarky comments. I was shocked that they would do this. I tried to remind myself that everyone needs a weekend away and just because I had a baby that didn't mean their lives had to stop. But why didn't they at least say something? I'm terrible at confrontations, so I ended up commenting HAVE FUN with no punctuation. *There,* I thought. *That will show them how upset I am!* As I said, I'm not good with confrontations.

The next morning, I had multiple notifications of messages in our group chat, but I couldn't bring myself to read them. I was sure they would say something along the lines of how they didn't want to be friends with me anymore and I wasn't ready to face that. I wanted to stay in this place where I didn't know exactly what was happening and I could pretend that everything was fine.

I eventually read the text messages and they were an endless string of things like WE MISS YOU and WISH YOU WERE WITH US! There were some references to me being there the next year, but there were no explanations as to why they hadn't told me they were going *this* year. More specifically, going without me. I got as close to a confrontation as I could by responding, I DIDN'T EVEN KNOW YOU WERE GOING. It wasn't very direct, but it got my message across.

WE KNEW YOU COULDN'T COME, read the reply. WE DIDN'T WANT YOU TO FEEL GUILTY OR TRY TO ACTUALLY GO AND LEAVE YOUR BABY, SO WE THOUGHT WE JUST WOULDN'T TELL YOU!

They were trying to be considerate of my feelings. And an exclamation point was used, which to me meant they were being kind. But I still felt unsettled. The remainder of the weekend was filled with texts from them saying they missed me, asking about my son, and declaring the weekend not as fun without me there. I appreciated their efforts, but it still made me feel sad and unsettled about my friendships I'd spent years nurturing.

EXPERT TIP

You may have some friends who seem quiet after your baby arrives, but that doesn't necessarily mean they are pulling away from you. In fact, what we often imagine in situations like this is far worse than reality. They could be giving you time and space to settle in with your baby or waiting to hear from you because they simply don't know what to do or how to approach you without feeling invasive. You're going to have to take the lead in some situations and address what's happening if it's troubling you. It's not always easy; sometimes it can actually feel scary because there is always a chance that the conversations can result in the end of the friendship. But it's better to know and begin to move forward, instead of living with tension or anxiety about the situation.

—Leslie Wasserman, LCSW

"It's inevitable that some people in your life are going to make assumptions about you once you become a parent to a newborn," says Leslie Wasserman, LCSW. "They presume that you won't be interested or have the time to do things you once did, and the calls, texts, and invitations will become less frequent or in some cases stop entirely."

In other words, some of your friendships will change after you have a baby.

This isn't an insult to the connection between you and those closest to you, and it doesn't mean that every relationship in your life will implode soon after you give birth. Some will actually grow stronger once your baby comes along. But it's an inevitable outcome that not everything will be the same after you undergo one of the biggest life changes, because you won't be the same, either.

As Wasserman explains it, "When you have a newborn baby, it is absolutely necessary to be consumed by your child because you are the person keeping them alive. Unfortunately, this may not align with where some of your friends are in that moment. It's no one's fault, but it is the reality of your situation."

This isn't meant to be a dire prognosis of what life will be like for you, and it doesn't mean giving birth will leave you with zero friends. Just that things can shift as you settle into your new reality. Please remember that you did nothing wrong, no one dislikes you, and this is not a situation unique to you. *All* new moms experience this in some form.

We resumed our group chat as usual the following week and I made a conscious effort not to talk about my son or motherhood and instead focus on them and their lives. And while they did occasionally ask me things in return, I noticed that it was generic pleasantries and nothing specific about my son's acid reflux or any of the things I'd told them about.

I started writing less and they didn't write to me, either. I had a million other things to do and putting effort toward relationships that felt almost superficial at this point was at the bottom of my list. We were in different places in our lives and somehow couldn't find anything to bridge the gap that was growing between us, and our group chat eventually became limited to birthday acknowledgments and holiday greetings. Our lives went in different directions and the things that once connected us started to matter less. It wasn't what I wanted to happen, but sometimes growing means growing apart from some of the people in your life.

One of the best things you can do is be up-front and honest with your friends in the early days or weeks of motherhood. Let them know your thoughts and feelings. If you're completely overwhelmed and exhausted, tell them. If phone calls give you anxiety, let people know. Everyone in your life wants you to be happy and healthy, to celebrate your new addition, and to continue being a good friend to you. But figuring out how to do all that—while also giving you the space you need right now—isn't an exact science.

You may feel as if some friends come on too strong while others may wait in silence for you to reach out when you can.

Many assumptions are often made to help fill in the blanks. And when we start substituting assumptions for facts, we stop communicating. Don't leave room for guessing; be up-front.

After months and months of avoiding calls and texts because I was so tired and depressed, then feeling guilty because I felt like I was single-handedly ruining my friendships, I wrote out one text and sent it to several people. I let everyone know that I'd been suffering from PPD, that I wasn't ignoring them, but I also wasn't quite ready to be fully present yet, either. The responses overwhelmed me: Everyone was incredibly understanding and supportive. I wish I'd texted everyone much sooner; it could have saved me a lot of sadness and guilt and spared my friends the worry and confusion they felt.

"Friendships should be flexible and able to weather storms," Wasserman notes. "There needs to be a give-and-take. Sometimes we can be more present than others and find our relationships easily fall back into place when we're able to be more engaged. And there are other times when people just aren't good friends and won't be there for you. But it takes a life change, like having a baby, for you to realize that. At a certain point, you have to ask yourself if the friendship is serving either of you. If it's not, you should consider focusing your efforts on other relationships instead, and move on."

I wish I didn't have to write this, but there is a possibility that one or more of your friendships will fade into acquaintances after your baby is born. While it's not exactly fun, this is the natural course of some friendships. People come in and out of our lives for a reason, and maybe what drew you together in the first place no longer exists or isn't that important to one or both of you anymore. It could be that you both loved dining out together, but you don't have time right now. And if that was the core of your connection, the relationship could potentially fade to black if you take that away.

Whatever the root cause may be, things between you are changing and the friendship might soon begin to feel as if it's run its course. I'm not saying this person will all but disappear from your world (although they may), but they might soon exist only as a face in your social media feed. It's okay, even healthy, to mourn the end of a friendship. But it's also important to remind yourself that there's always a chance that you and this person might reconnect at some point down the road.

Part of my job over the seven or eight months before my son was born was to document my pregnancy for a global parenting website. Through that, I connected with several women who reached out to me who were also first-time mothers, all due within a few months of one another. I'd grown close with them during my pregnancy and had come to rely on and *need* the support and camaraderie we shared.

I had plenty of existing friends who were also moms, and they, too, were a source of help and support. But there is something special about someone who is going through the same thing as you are in the same moment. We were in the trenches together, side by side, as we endured diaper blowouts, communication struggles with our partners, and leaky breasts. Yes, many of my other friends knew all about those things, but memories become hazy with time. Other friends didn't have kids yet (or never planned to), and they had no way to truly grasp the massive impact my new baby was having on my life. But these women knew exactly what I was going through and how it felt because they were all living it along with me.

I clung to them, and our communication was endless. And there was something about us all being in the same exhausted and hormonally charged headspace that made it easy to go from talking about the benefits of hemorrhoid cream versus gel to our favorite TV shows or future life plans. In short, all the conversations I'd once had with multiple people were now happening within a very small group of people.

Just be aware that the people in your life may not be as enthusiastic as you are about your new virtual friendships. They may feel replaced, or that you're turning to strangers instead of them. Keep reminding them that this is a connection you need in addition to what you have with them, not in lieu of it. And that connecting with another mom who is in the same stage as you can be a lifeline right now.

I also experienced some surprises along the way—things I never would have guessed would happen. Friends I wasn't necessarily

Real Mom Story

In a bizarre coincidence, I was pregnant at the same time as two other friends, and our babies were all due within a few months of each other. We all grew much closer during our pregnancies. I was the second of us to give birth and I immediately struggled. My daughter was not an easy baby, by any means, and I was surprised that my friend who gave birth first didn't mention just how hard it was. By the time my third friend gave birth a few months after me, I felt so broken by motherhood that I was worried for her sanity. I dropped off several frozen meals from my own stash and made a point to check on her frequently. To my surprise, she said motherhood was easier than she expected. And our other friend agreed! I felt like I was doing something wrong. It became clear that just as pregnancy drew us closer, motherhood divided us. They didn't want to hear my problems. I never expected an event that seemed like it was going to bond us for a lifetime would be the reason our friendship eventually ended.

—Kara G.

that close with became some of my closest confidants. There is something about motherhood that allows you to let your guard down and be vulnerable. And sometimes when two mothers are willing to be equally vulnerable, they connect—and a bond grows quickly. These were some of the women who listened to me, endorsed my feelings as real and valid, gave me a safe space to be honest, and shared their unfiltered stories of motherhood in return.

Yes, there were some friendships that struggled. Maybe we just couldn't be what the other needed in that moment, and that's okay. Things change and people grow. I was fortunate that most of the distance was seasonal and existed just for this particular period of time in my life. As my son grew older and I stepped out of the fog of PPD, we were able to reconnect.

I also learned that some of my friends, while wonderful and loving, just aren't "baby" people. They would have been there in a heartbeat if I needed them, but they didn't have a strong presence in my first year of motherhood because it was completely foreign to them. Interestingly enough, most of these people are actually "kid" people—meaning they are much more comfortable with kids than babies—and are now some of my son's most treasured "family."

To better understand why some friendships will feel the strain of your new role in life while others continue unaffected—or become even stronger—it helps to recognize where your friends are in their lives right now and how that fits in with your impending new arrival.

While there is no way to encapsulate every friendship, in my experience I noticed that my friends generally fell into one of four categories. This is not to say that everyone in your world will fit perfectly into these groups, because each of us is different and every friendship is unique. But I'm going to paint with a broad brush just for a moment so that we can examine what stage everyone in your life will be in when your new baby arrives, and how that might factor into your postpartum friendships.

Friends with younger kids. This will generally be your sweet spot. These friends are either actively dealing with the same things you are, or at least they were doing it recently enough to remember how hard things may be for you right now.

Friends with older kids. You may automatically assume they will be understanding if you need to cut an outing short to get your baby home for a nap, but that won't always be the case. Yes, they are also parents, but not *new* parents. The passage of time can cloud our memories, and, to put it plainly, many veteran parents forget how hard it actually is and think some new parents are a bit overdramatic.

Friends without kids who may want kids one day. This group can go either way. Yes, they have a personal interest in what you are going through, which can lead them to be very engaged with you during this time. But that may also backfire. Some future

---

EXPERT TIP

Many women find themselves feeling isolated in early motherhood. They are so busy taking care of their baby that they don't have time for much else, and understandably so. But it can be hard to know how to reconnect with people once life becomes more manageable. Ideally, the onus shouldn't be on you, but the reality is that it usually is. I recommend starting slowly, so you don't feel overwhelmed. Reach out to one friend and tell them how you're feeling, specifically one of the friends you know can and will want to help. It's also a good idea to take stock of your relationships during your pregnancy. If you are already feeling disconnected from some people, you might want to pay extra attention to that relationship. Think of it like taking prenatal vitamins for your friendships. What you're doing now will make things better when your baby is born.

—Leslie Wasserman, LCSW

---

parents closely observe parents, and often form opinions of how they would handle a situation, or how well their nonexistent babies will sleep. And, of course, their imaginary babies will be easier to handle than the real one currently screaming in your arms as you try to have an adult conversation. Many keep those opinions to themselves, but you might be faced with some silent judgment and unsolicited advice. Specifically, advice on how to be a better parent from a person who isn't a parent yet.

Friends who are trying to conceive or aren't able to conceive. These friends are going through a lot, some—or even all—of which you may not be aware of. I struggled to conceive for quite some time and can vividly recall the bitter-sweet feeling upon hearing friend after friend announce their pregnancy. I was happy for them, but it also shined a spotlight on my inability to do what seemed to come so easily to every-one else. I would smile, congratulate them, and sometimes go home and cry. I'd often wrestle with the guilt I felt over my sadness or jealousy. If this person is a close friend, you probably know what they have been dealing with and will be under-standing and supportive of any reaction they might have. "It's important to validate someone in this situation," Wasserman advises. "Let them have their space but also make sure they know you are there. Pregnancy announcements can be very triggering for anyone who has suffered a pregnancy loss or is facing infertility."

It may be hard to fathom, but within a year of the birth of your baby, you will have new friends in your life. And that will continue happening as your child enters preschool or elemen-tary school and starts playing sports or pursuing other activities. Children open up an entirely new world for us, and through everything they do, you will be exposed to other parents, some of whom will become your true friends. This doesn't mean that you'll be replacing everyone in your life in favor of other parents of similarly aged children. It's just a reminder of the ever-evolving life circumstances that will impact your friendships.

Some of your friends may not understand the magnitude of the shift in your universe. Relationships will evolve, but that doesn't mean they all need to end. I struggled with these changes and felt immense (and unnecessary) guilt for far too long. I don't want you to take time away from your baby because you are worried about your friends.

It won't all be easy and there will be growing pains. But there is also the possibility of existing friendships growing stronger and new friends entering your life. I can't tell you how to preserve every relationship so that it stays as is, but I do know this: After the initial shakeup, all the pieces land exactly where they are meant to be. And the people around you will both nurture and support your new role in life.

Now, I don't want this to seem like canned advice or one of those awful motivational quotes that inspire no one, so I've written some very specific things to help you through all this.

1. Shifts in friendships can't be avoided.

No matter how positive you may be that your friendships will remain completely unchanged after you welcome your baby, it's still going to happen. Because you will change. Not every relationship will be affected, and it won't necessarily be all bad. But it will happen. And in the end, you'll be better because of it.

Real Mom Story

I was the first among my friend group to have a baby. Only one relationship changed after my son was born—and it happened to be with my best friend. Before I gave birth, we talked daily and she even hosted my baby shower. But once my son was born, I stopped hearing from her. I'll admit that I didn't reach out as often as I used to, but my free time was very limited in those early months. She had only seen my son a few times and had no interest in holding him, which made me sad. I tried to give her space and would reach out when I could to say hello, but our conversations were brief and awkward. As my son got older, I tried even harder to reconnect, but it was useless. Our relationship isn't the same and I don't think she wants it to be. I want to ask if I did something wrong, but I honestly don't know where to begin. I wondered if she was going through something and didn't want to discuss it. But I also couldn't keep fighting for something one-sided; I needed to put that time and effort into friendships that were mutual and supportive. If you do find yourself in that situation, maybe it's time to reconsider who your friends are.

—Jen B.

2. It's really not you. Or them.

The changes won't occur because someone said or did anything, but because a bigger event—in this case, the birth of your baby—has completely changed your world. You didn't cause this, and they didn't, either. It happens to everyone to one degree or another and there is nothing different or wrong with you. Remember: This is a huge life change, and it will impact every aspect of your life. Including your friendships.

3. You need to be honest. And remember that they might not know how to proceed.

Please don't assume that the people in your world will know exactly how to approach you. In some cases, they might be waiting to follow your lead and that's why you're not hearing from them. Or they overwhelm you with their attempted involvement. People will do what they think is the best course of action until you tell them otherwise. Be up-front with your friends about your feelings and needs. It's okay to make this about you in the beginning.

4. It's okay to prioritize your online friends.

Things like social media and virtual mom groups may introduce you to new friends, specifically other moms who are experiencing the same things you are. Don't downplay the significance of these relationships in your life at this time. Embrace these connections. It's wonderful to have someone to talk with who is also going through the same thing as you.

5. Children will continuously bring new people into your life.

Whether you find the majority of your friendships faltering or only just a few, you'll repeatedly make new friends through your child. This is not to say that you will swap everyone in your life for fellow parents; it's just a reminder that while motherhood can change some friendships, it will also bring many new ones into your life as well.

6. Your baby has changed your life, not theirs.

It can be very easy to get caught up in your new baby and relish every moment, big or small. And it's normal to want to share all of that with those closest to you. Just remember that, while this is a massive and exciting new addition to your life, the impact isn't the same for your friends. And they might not share your feelings of pure elation when looking at a photo of your baby. Don't take it personally. It doesn't mean that they don't care about you or your baby. But the significance of everything your child does will always be greater for you than for anyone else. Except maybe some grandparents.

Real Mom Story

I had a close group of friends during law school, and it stayed that way for a number of years afterward; we'd regularly get together at least once a month. But as soon as I announced my pregnancy, I started being left out of group messages and not told when they were getting together. I tried to stay connected, but was told things like, "We're going to stay out late—you'll be tired" or "You can't even drink right now." Not one of them even contacted me after my son was born. I've thought about this (and overthought it, I'm sure) and realized that there are ages and stages to friendships. You have school friendships that may end when you graduate. Work friendships that only last while you're in the same office. And you'll be continuously making new mom friends based on the ages of your children and their activities. It's wonderful when you make a friendship that lasts beyond your common bonds, but I think we assume that is always going to be the rule when it's more likely the exception. Life changes will change your friendships. And becoming a mom is a big change.

—Isabelle W.

7. This could be hard for them.

It doesn't matter if you've been diagnosed with infertility or had minimal struggles trying to conceive. We all know how hard it can be to see others getting pregnant and welcoming new babies when we're still waiting. And I don't care what anyone says about always taking the high road: We can be envious or even resent those closest to us who seem to have zero problems in this area. If a friend is acting strangely, or seems to be avoiding you, give them the benefit of the doubt. We never truly know what someone else is feeling or going through. Seeing and hearing about your baby may be too painful for them right now, even if they already have children. When one of my best friends told me about her pregnancy, I broke down in tears that were a combination of happiness for her and heartbreak for me. Feelings can be complicated and confusing.

8. Some friendships might grow into something you never expected.

Motherhood can be a great connector. And while that doesn't mean you'll automatically befriend anyone with a child, you will find that it strengthens some of your already existing friendships. People who may have been on the periphery of your life at one point can grow into trusted confidants as you bond over being a mom.

Real Mom Story

A casual friend and I both shared on social media that we were pregnant and expecting a couple months apart. It led us to meet for lunch, and we became true friends. When our babies were born, we had regular playdates, long phone conversations, couples' nights out, late-night texts of encouragement, and she and her husband were our daughter's godparents. Strangely enough, both babies were diagnosed with the same severe food allergy. It was comforting for me to be closely bonded to another mother who was experiencing the same challenges, and it made playdates and dinners out easier.

Our daughter was thriving with our lifestyle and medical changes; her son was not. Our daughter began gaining weight where her son had to have a feeding tube inserted. We remained close, but I could feel tension building. Playdates were canceled or postponed, texts went unanswered, and those encouraging phone conversations were nonexistent. But I held out hope. It is so easy to get trapped in comparisons as a mother. I don't blame her, but I miss her tremendously.

We all experience motherhood differently and can't manage how our actions are interpreted by others. If a relationship that has ended isn't toxic, we need to keep an open heart.

—Diana H.

9. Some friendships will end.

This doesn't mean there will be a falling-out, or that you'll have disdain for one another. Rather, you'll start to notice that the friendship is no longer serving either one of you. And that's okay; you've just gone through a life upheaval and your world is different. Be grateful for the friendship you shared and focus on how important it was to you at one time, instead of dwelling on the now.

10. This is all part of the natural evolution of relationships, and completely common among new moms.

If you look back over your life, you'll realize that several of your relationships have ebbed and flowed throughout the years, and some have ended. This isn't the first time you've had friendships change or even end, though you may feel the weight of it more so now than ever before. It can feel especially massive because it's happening along with so many other changes in your life right now and possibly with more than one person. It's similar to postpartum hair loss in a way. It's a natural cycle that's transpired before, only this time there might be a lot of it happening all at the same time.

CHAPTER 12
Finding Childcare

Mary Poppins isn't available.

Moms are often complimented for their multitasking skills, praised for their abilities to seemingly be able to "do it all." But why do we *need* to do everything ourselves? It's become commonplace to refer to moms as superheroes, frame it as a huge compliment, and let the narrative continue.

I say that it's time to change the script.

The days of the superhero mother, the woman who is being run into the ground as she tries to do it all because "that's what moms do," are over. We need and deserve help. And that includes childcare.

There are many reasons you may need help—and all are valid. You could be going back to work. Or maybe you work from home. You could just need help because caring for a new baby is hard enough in itself, let alone everything else you're already doing. It doesn't matter *why* a mom needs childcare (and remember, you don't have to justify your decision to anyone); the road to finding a caregiver for your new baby—and the feelings that will accompany you once you do—is often intense.

Breaking a stigma that has existed for generations isn't easy. You'll be fighting internal feelings of guilt while possibly facing external judgments. It's important to remember why you are hiring help, and if being called "selfish" means you're prioritizing yourself *and* your child, I say wear that as a badge of honor. You're doing it right. Your child needs a happy and healthy mom.

This concept of moms valuing themselves and their children at the same time is slowly starting to take hold, and, frankly, it's about time. One approach that more and more moms have been sharing with me lately is women who work just to pay for childcare. What they earn is about equal to what they pay, but they *want* to work. They enjoy it, are passionate about their careers, and find themselves happier and more fulfilled—and therefore, in their case, a better parent—when they work.

Until I became a mom myself, my personal experience with childcare began and ended with the babysitting I did in high school. I had no real knowledge of the range of services that could be included with certain types of childcare, and you shouldn't feel that you're behind the curve if you don't, either. After all, it wasn't until I became a mom that I even considered the fact that sanitizing a breast pump's tubes would be an item on my to-do list, let alone something I could have someone help with.

I was working from home long before it became a pandemic cliché, and my husband and I planned for me to continue doing that after our son was born. I'd be cutting back my hours to accommodate my other "job" of being our son's sole caregiver while my husband was at his office. We assumed it was a foolproof plan.

We were wrong. He and I indeed were the fools, and we crumbled under the weight of our plan. In hindsight, we really didn't put much thought into it at all. It was more like, "I'm already home, so there's no reason why the baby can't be here with me as I work. Problem solved!" Unfortunately, there were *many* reasons that it wasn't a great idea, but we didn't bother to consider any of them.

That's not to say we didn't have some things that worked in our favor. I had deadlines for writing assignments, but it was up to me to decide when to do the actual writing. I wasn't beholden to a typical 9 a.m.–5 p.m. work schedule, which provided the necessary flexibility to even attempt to do this. Also, I worked for a team of mothers at a parenting website. If anyone would understand why I might be late for a meeting due to a diaper blowout or be able to tune out the sound of my breast pump during a phone call (which happened more than once), it was this group of incredibly supportive and understanding people. And I recognize how lucky I was because of that.

Even with all the things that were in my favor, there still comes a specific point when work must be done. And a baby must be fed. Or changed, bathed, comforted, burped, etc. And it was when these two "jobs" of mine intersected, which they did frequently, that I began having problems.

EXPERT TIP

Before you even arrive at the interview stage, you should have a solid list prepared of what responsibilities you hope this person or facility will take on. While you can expect similar providers to offer generally the same terms of service, the exact scope of work is specific to each one. It never hurts to ask for extras. Just be aware that you may have to pay more. And be realistic with your asks. Most importantly, have a written contract of the scope of work you've both agreed upon; otherwise, you run the risk of one party feeling dissatisfied or even being taken advantage of.

—Marquis Anne, childcare expert

I found myself with only little snippets of time during the day when I could walk away from my son in his bassinet and write. I would just be starting to find a rhythm, and I'd be summoned away by my other boss. Trying to write, research, or conduct an interview in fits and starts was proving nearly impossible. I began waiting to work until my husband came home, but I was often so tired by then that it would take twice as long to get anything done.

Next, I tried to bundle my assignments, and, instead of turning them in one at a time, I'd wait until my parents came to visit to get them all done. A good idea, but I was still tired and had to stop to breastfeed or pump. Still, it was the best scenario, and I was able to get my work done during daylight hours. Unfortunately, my parents weren't going to move in with us to accommodate my work schedule, and we needed another plan.

We considered our options and decided that a mother's helper would best fit our needs. Although it shares the same name, this type of mother's helper is different from the one favored by housewives in the 1960s to help deal with stress and anxiety. *That* mother's helper was known as "benzos," aka benzodiazepines, a class of drugs that produce sedation and relieve anxiety. The kind I was interested in wasn't addictive.

Unlike a nanny or day care, a mother's helper isn't solely responsible for a child and instead helps around the house and with the baby while the mother is *also* at home—and is a much more affordable option. A former coworker hired her teenage niece as her mother's helper, and a friend enlisted a trusted neighbor to work as her helper. We were still new to the area, so we looked into finding someone through an agency.

Unfortunately, things never progressed beyond that. Once word of our plan began to circulate among the people in our lives, the feedback began rolling in. And it wasn't good.

It ranged from pity that I "couldn't handle things" to outright disgust that I would even consider having help when I was home all day. I wish I could say I ignored it all and proceeded with the plan, but I didn't. I felt guilty and was ashamed of myself, and the thoughts of how "everyone but me can handle this" intensified. Essentially, I let the opinions of others shape my decision and didn't hire help. Instead, I did that detrimental thing that moms often do; I sucked it up and kept going, even though I shouldn't have. But that's what we moms do, right?

If any form of childcare can help you, and is accessible, I implore you to utilize—or at least strongly consider—it before dismissing the idea as something you think you don't need. Whether it's paying for a professional or just having a family member or friend step in occasionally, there is no law that says you have to be the primary caregiver the majority of the time. Keep in mind that it's healthy for you not to always be on high alert and let your mind rest.

There are myriad childcare options, ranging from the more common choices of day care and nannies to a more personalized approach, including nanny shares and childcare swaps. Each has its benefits, and the pros and cons will be different for each family because not everyone has the same needs. This is why it's important for you to take the time to think about your wants and expectations from childcare. Do you need more flexibility with your hours? Is it important for your child's caregiver to also introduce them to a particular educational curriculum? These are just a couple considerations to keep in mind. On page 297, I've compiled a list of questions to ask when you're considering childcare options, which should help steer you toward one option as opposed to another.

Cost is obviously a leading factor in selecting childcare, and it isn't as easy to approximate as you might think. Marquis Anne, childcare and caregiver expert, and founder of Nanny Village, a family staffing agency, told me that the national average cost for childcare is around $10,500 per child annually, according to recent reports. "But it's just not realistic to consider a number like this because there are so many personal factors that will affect your specific costs, such as where you live, the age of your kids, and how many children you have," says Anne. "Not to mention the type of care you select, the experience level and education of your caregiver, and their scope of duties—these will all factor into your overall costs. I've worked with clients who turned to family or friends for childcare, which can be free in some cases, to others who've spent more than $100,000 a year for a live-in nanny with extensive experience."

Once you've identified your budget and initial needs, you can begin to focus on what type of childcare will best suit your family. And, by doing this initial work, the rest of the process will go much more smoothly. You may be able to eliminate certain categories of caregivers because they won't be compatible with your work schedule or budget. You'll have everything you want—and don't want—clearly outlined, which can then be used as your interview questions. And you'll know where to begin your search, which may include personal referrals, agencies, and caregiving websites.

Real Mom Story

When I became pregnant with my son, my husband and I found a day care we loved—and could afford—but knew we might have a problem some days with their non-negotiable pickup time. We asked my mother-in-law, who lived nearby and worked part-time, if she might be able to help.

"I can do even better than that," she said. "I was planning to retire next year, but I'd rather do it now . . . and be your nanny! Free of charge, of course."

We didn't even make it one week without friction.

My son was having some nipple confusion as he adjusted to the bottle, so my pediatrician recommended not using a pacifier. But, unbeknownst to us, my mother-in-law went out and bought him every pacifier ever made until she found one that he would use. By day three he refused to latch and would only take the bottle. And his pacifier.

We eventually had to end the arrangement and send our son to the day care we'd originally planned on. It completely fractured our relationship with my husband's parents.

In hindsight, I wish I'd never accepted her offer. We should have agreed on everything beforehand and paid her even a little something so that we didn't feel so indebted.

—Valerie C.

Researching childcare options brings with it a whole new confusing vocabulary. Some of the options sound the same but aren't. Knowing what the service calls itself can help you determine your expectations and also what questions to ask.

Day care: A facility with a structured program for a group of children who are typically same-aged peers. A day care must be licensed and follow specific state-mandated protocols. Many day cares are local franchisees of a larger, national organization. Typically, this will cost less than a nanny, but the hours will be less flexible, and protocols and policies more rigid. However, with several caregivers on staff, parents aren't reliant on finding backup care if someone calls in sick.

In-home day care: A similar structure to a day-care facility, but in the caregiver's home. They also must meet strict licensing standards. While a residential program can be more affordable than a day-care facility and have a lower caregiver-to-student ratio, with a smaller group of children, your child might have less of a same-aged peer group.

Nanny: An individual providing personalized, ongoing care in your home (or another designated home), specific to your family and your child's needs. You'll be paying a higher cost and be responsible for alternate care when your nanny is sick or taking a day off. However, as the sole employer, you can enjoy more flexibility and be able to dictate the overall structure.

Nanny share: An individual care provider working for more than one family (typically only two). The nanny and children usually alternate weekly between homes. While the cost can be more for multiple children, it's overall more affordable because the families split the cost. However, the care will not be one-on-one, and the structure will need to be mutually agreed-upon by you and the other family.

Babysitter: An on-call caregiver a family hires sporadically for short periods of time.

Au pair: A young adult from another country who will live with your family on a legal visa, generally for a two-year contract. In exchange for payment, room, and board, they will provide in-home care. They can sometimes provide your child and family with new cultural experiences. Due to the complex paperwork, an au pair should be hired through a licensed agency. This option best serves families who need childcare outside of normal hours.

Care swap: An arrangement between you and another family (generally friends, relatives, or close acquaintances) to take turns providing care for one another. This works well if you have complementary work schedules (usually part-time), or both need occasional care.

Family or friend: A trusted family member or friend who is available and capable of providing childcare. Although this is often offered for little to no money, consider some form of compensation and a contract outlining your needs, parenting philosophies, and safety protocols.

Mother's helper: This person essentially assists the mother at home with any needs related to the household or the baby. It can range from light housework to playing with a baby while the mother takes a shower, works, takes a break, or does whatever she may need to do. A mother's helper is not a sole caregiver and works *while* the mom is also in the house.

Family assistant: This person will help with any or every need your family has, such as running errands, walking your dog, managing household needs, stocking the refrigerator, meal prep, or light housework. While they can occasionally help with babysitting or driving children to and from school or activities, their primary responsibility is not childcare. The specific job details will be outlined on a case-by-case basis. Some families will begin working with their nanny before their baby is born by having them start as a family assistant, allowing them to both get to know one another and introducing the nanny to the family's routine ahead of the new arrival.

Travel nanny: A travel nanny is someone who accompanies a family on trips and provides typical nanny services in a different location. A travel nanny can be used if your family's nanny or caregiver is unable to accompany you on a trip, or if you need short-term care in a different location. In addition to payment, you will be required to pay cost of travel, provide food, and generally offer a private bedroom and per diem compensation.

If you are wondering where to begin this search, you have a few options for how to approach this. All of these are equally good methods, and the one you choose will depend on your personal preference.

A complete DIY approach: Create a list of your care needs and determine what options best fit your family. Seek out potential facilities through research and recommendations. Ask your friends or family, and seek referrals from your local moms group on Facebook. Curate a list of leads and then begin the interview and background process on your own.

Care finder website: These sites, such as Winnie.com for pre-school day care and Care.com for all types of caregivers, offer services somewhere in between doing it all yourself and hiring an agency. You will likely pay a small fee and be guided through the process, but there won't be the handholding and personal assistance you would find through an agency. You should also expect to perform background checks yourself in addition to checking references.

Staffing agency: The most thorough of services, an agency will essentially handhold you through this process. You'll pay a fee and they will do the legwork for you, essentially delivering a list of handpicked and prescreened options for your review and consideration.

EXPERT TIP

Waiting lists for day care are a real thing. Layoffs and facility closures during the pandemic have left us with a shortage of childcare providers. I recommend starting to evaluate your childcare needs and looking into options early in your pregnancy because we have been seeing waiting lists of up to one year for a day-care facility. It can also take that long to find the right nanny for your family because the workforce is so depleted. Start early!

—Marquis Anne

You also must take into account all your needs, both on a daily basis and in special circumstances, which can range from anything such as a child's food allergies to the occasional late pickup. To help you further narrow down your options, I've curated a list of possible needs for you to consider, based on conversations I've had with many moms over the past few years. Keep in mind that, while this includes what has been most frequently shared with me, you might have some questions that are even more niche. After all, I once watched a nanny interview unfold on an episode of *The Real Housewives of New York City* where the candidate was asked if she would stand in line at sample sales or "do blowouts" on the mother's hair. We all have different needs and budgets, I guess.

You may decide to return to work once you've secured childcare. Whether you find yourself dreading this day or counting down the hours until you strip off your mom jeans and jump headfirst into the workplace, the transition back into this segment of your pre-baby life as a new mom won't be without hiccups.

Aside from adjusting to being apart from your baby, you may have to manage the expectations of your supervisor or coworkers. Many nonparents (and some veteran ones as well) don't understand all that maternity leave entails and will treat your return as if you were off on a paid vacation. There could be tension from colleagues who resent you for leaving work at a set time each day to relieve your childcare instead of staying at the office all hours of the night—or joining the team for happy hour. Add in the possibility that you may need to find a place in the office to pump between meetings, and you will likely find yourself realizing that this process is more emotionally draining than you imagined it would be.

Try to remind yourself that you have every right to set boundaries. It will take time to adjust to being a working mom, for both you and your colleagues. The most important thing you can do is communicate. Be honest and up-front, ask for flexibility, and make your needs known. Don't expect to have it all figured out by day one; many moms report this transition can take anywhere from a few weeks to months until everything is ironed out. Enlist the support of your partner, family, and friends while you navigate this situation.

Choosing a caregiver for your child will undoubtedly be one of the most painstaking and important decisions you'll make as a new parent, likely leaving you feeling overwhelmed and second-guessing yourself. It's okay to admit that; in fact, it's good to be honest with yourself and your caregiver about your feelings. You aren't the first parent to be worried about leaving your child in the care of someone else, and your caregiver likely has experienced this before and can help address your concerns.

As parents, we know our children best and it's hard to imagine anyone else being qualified to care for them as we do. But remember: You aren't looking to replace yourself entirely, but rather hiring the next best thing to you. Your childcare provider can and will become a trusted member of your community in time. And just because Mary Poppins is likely retired by now—and also she's a fictional character—that doesn't mean you won't find someone equally well suited to your needs. Just don't expect them to always be singing or carry a magic carpetbag. At any rate, here are a few super-califragilisticexpialidocious points that I want you to remember when you begin your search.

1. Let go of the guilt. Or at least try to feel *less* guilty.

This is always easier said than done, I know. And, yes, you will feel guilt, you will worry and wonder what your child is doing each and every second you are apart. That is completely natural and common and will lessen over time. If you can, visit your child on your lunch break, start work late one day, or leave a little early. Breaks like that will help you ease into your new routine.

2. This is your child. This is a time when you can and should be a mama bear.

Don't feel that you are being too careful during your research, because that's impossible. This is your child. Ask to see licenses and certifications. Collect as many references as possible and call them. Ask around in mom groups and on social media for reviews. Request background checks and fingerprints and pay for professional background checks if you have to. This decision is about who you will entrust with your child's care. There is no such thing as too much research.

3. You don't have to work full-time to hire help.

There is no law that says you must work a forty-hour week in order to enlist help. You don't even have to work at all. Don't try to do it all because it's absolutely impossible. Something will suffer, and it will likely be you. And, if someone in your life has a problem with that, give them a key to your house so they don't have to break in when they come over to do your laundry and all the other tasks you don't have time to tackle because you are busy keeping a tiny baby alive.

4. Nothing is free.

A common form of childcare is having a family member or friend watch your child, which is often provided by the person at no cost. While this is a generous offer, you should still create a contract or written agreement so that nothing is left to chance. Otherwise, if left to proceed as an informal arrangement, you might find yourself with little say because this other person is doing you a favor. Compensate them in any way you can, whether that is a small amount of money each month, gift cards, or doing a favor in return.

EXPERT TIP

If you are hiring an individual caregiver, I always recommend paying them through an official payroll company, as opposed to trying to do it yourself. Not only is it helpful to have an impartial third party managing payment and records, but they will take care of everything—from handling time off and holiday pay to withholding taxes. Plus, you can take advantage of a federal caregiver tax credit.

—Marquis Anne

---

5. Always have a backup plan. And a backup to that.

It's inevitable that your childcare will become unexpectedly unavailable one day, and that reason could be because your nanny is sick, your child is too sick to go to day care, or any other type of unplanned reason or emergency on either side. This isn't always going to be something that comes with ample warning; you may be faced with this situation just as you are about to leave the house or during the middle of a workday. Identify who will be able to stay home with your child in the event that you won't be able to utilize day care. You need to work out a solid backup plan as an initial step to this entire process. And remember: Emergencies don't wait for a convenient time. It's entirely possible that your backup plan's availability might not always match your needs. Yes, that means you will need a backup to your backup.

6. It never hurts to ask for something ahead of time.

Maybe you actually do want a caregiver who will stand in line for you at sample sales or teach your child Klingon. You will never know if that's even a possibility until you ask. Be honest and up-front with your wants and needs, but also be respectful. This person's primary role and responsibility is to care for your child, something they are highly qualified to do, and you don't want to treat them as your personal assistant. Agree on any extras ahead of time and include them in your contract. And pay extra because you are likely asking for work outside the general scope of duties for this position.

7. Have a trial period.

This is your child. *Your child.* You want to be as sure as possible that your chosen caregiver is a match for your family. And you should also want that person to be sure that you match them as well and that they are excited to care for your baby. The best way to be sure of this is through a paid trial period, which should be a mutually agreed-upon amount of time (minimum one week) when both sides test out the arrangement. Afterward, each party can decide if they want to move forward. And, yes, you run the risk of the caregiver deciding it's not a fit for them and having to go back to the interview stage or calling on your second choice. But you also have the same option and can end a situation that doesn't work for you before you are contractually liable.

Real Mom Story

When my son was first born, we hired a babysitter who had just finished nursing school and was also working part-time at a nearby pediatric eye and ear institute. It was clear how much she loved him. One evening we came home early and found her introducing him to her parents over FaceTime. As a mom, it made my heart so happy to see how much he meant to her.

When he was around two years old, he had surgery at her hospital. She changed her entire schedule around so that she could be with him in recovery, and he would be able to wake up to a familiar face. When we finally were able to go to his room, we found him in her arms in a rocking chair, completely peaceful and content.

I still get choked up when I picture her holding him. I was a nervous wreck about him going under anesthesia and then coming out of it, and she eased all of my worries by assuring me that she would be there with him when I wasn't able to. She showed me that there are indeed people out there who will love your kids almost as much as you do.

—Avery P.

8. Keep the lines of communication open.

There can never be too many questions when it comes to your child. Decide on a check-in schedule and make sure it's included in your contract. And don't be afraid to ask questions or raise concerns at other times. Constant communication can help offset challenges before they even arise, because you aren't just waiting to talk until there is a full-blown problem. Again, this is your child. Ask away.

9. Be a good employer.

Remember: Even if you are paying through an agency or billing service and not directly writing a check to your nanny or the individual staff at your day care, you are still the employer. And just as you want the best possible caregiver for your child, that person wants to work for the best possible boss. Treat this person or persons with the respect they deserve. Consider providing your nanny with meals if they are with your child during the workday. Or perhaps you can give coffee gift cards to the day-care staff (even if it's $5, the gesture is what matters) or surprise your nanny with a bonus day off. Recognize them on birthdays and holidays with a card or, when your child gets older, a handmade card. One day, I collected the dirty towels and rags at my son's preschool and took them home to wash and fold. His teacher told me it had been a nagging item on her to-do list and the small gesture made a big impact. It doesn't always have to be a monetary gift; simply letting these people know you recognize, respect, and appreciate them can make a big difference.

CONCLUSION

Your New Normal

Welcome to Oz, Dorothy. Your world will now be in color.

I sat on a bench outside the Mommy & Me class I'd been taking with my nearly one-year-old son and cried. Okay, it was more like sobbing. The ugly kind where your face turns bright red. Snot oozed out my nose and mixed with tears; it probably looked like I had snail trails running down my cheeks. I tried to talk, but all that came out was a dramatic gasp for air in between a poor attempt at trying to string enough words together to form a sentence.

My friend was seated next to me and held my hand while patiently waiting for me to compose myself as our sons toddled around where we were seated, distracted from my hysterics by some leaves they'd found on the ground. Eventually, I was able to calm down, wipe my eyes and snotty nose, and speak.

"I'm finally a mom," I explained. "Well, not *finally*. But sometimes it overwhelms me."

I continued to explain. Our class had done an art project with our kids that day. It was their handprint inside a heart, very basic. But when I collected mine to take home and saw my son's name on it, all I could think was that I'm a mom. *A mom!* After all these years of being on the sidelines and watching my family and friends experience this, it was now my turn. I would be the one who would have these sweet yet often unidentifiable art projects from my child hanging on my refrigerator. It was everything I'd wanted for so long, and that red handprint on a piece of wrinkled paper served as a reminder that I was finally where I'd always wanted to be.

Becoming a parent is a lot like Dorothy's journey in *The Wizard of Oz*. You're naively going about your life until one day the skies darken, and a tornado blows into town. You think you're as prepared for this event as you could possibly be. You built the storm cellar and stocked it with supplies, but the tornado is more powerful than you anticipated. It picks up everything in its path, spins it around in its vortex, and spits it all back out—only nothing lands where it once was.

Everything around you is black and hazy in the wake of that tornado. And in the early days of new parenthood as well. There is a casual theory shared among moms called the "One Hundred Days of Darkness." The idea is that the first three months (technically 3.2 months) with a new baby are the hardest because you're in a fog, living only to be a servant to this tiny dictator who loves to scream. But, the idea holds, the magic three-month mark begins the ending to all that. Babies are able to sleep more, and they become more engaged and less fussy. Moms are more confident in their caregiving skills and are better adjusted to all the changes motherhood brings.

Hearing about this gave me hope. *Okay,* I thought. *One hundred days. Three months. That is the light at the end of the tunnel.* Maybe I would have to squint to be able to see it now in the distance, but before long it would be bright and right in front of me. At last, I had a time frame for when I could expect the aftereffects of this tornado to begin to dissipate. And a goal of hanging on until then.

I didn't think everything would be perfect by day 101, but I had high hopes that it would be considerably better. It actually is—for some people, that is. I still struggled beyond that date, which is also common. However, instead of recognizing that I might have PPD or that my son was just a really poor sleeper, I simply went back to my original thought: I would feel this way forever. I was wrong.

I didn't know that then. But I do now. And you have the advantage of all my hindsight right in front of you. It *will* get better. Unfortunately, there is no set date or timeline you can follow because it's different for everyone. But I can promise you that, long before your baby's first birthday, sunny skies will eventually replace the devastation left by that tornado.

With each day that passes, the world around you will grow brighter. And as you adjust your eyes to the light, you'll begin to realize that the tornado didn't actually cause destruction after all. It changed some things, sure. But it also blew away all that darkness and, for the first time, everything is in color.

As you further explore the post-tornado world, you might notice that it left you with some gifts, too—or did you have them all along?

You have *brains*. You learned so much about yourself, your relationship, and caring for a baby. You also have *courage*. You recognized just how strong you actually are after enduring childbirth and the struggles of being a new parent, and your confidence soared. Of course, you have a *heart*. You've seen that it has opened wider and is capable of loving more than you ever thought possible. And, just like Dorothy, you have finally found your way home and are settling into your new life as a mother.

But by the end of that first year, you will be parenting a completely different child than the tiny newborn you were first introduced to. Your baby will be crawling or even walking, and you'll be busy babyproofing your home. Their personality will develop quickly, and they might even be saying a few words. For me, this was when parenting truly became enjoyable. My son was funny, engaged, and developing from that helpless baby into a talking, walking, and laughing little boy.

Yes, the first year is harder than you could imagine and the lows are pretty far down there. But the highs are like nothing you can imagine. The first time your child smiles, laughs, or reaches for you is like nothing else.

Motherhood does change you—it's impossible for it not to. But that's not a bad thing. So many people try to fight this concept or tell you that you need to remain the person you were before the baby. To me, that makes no sense. We need to evolve and have a life that allows room for our child, our relationships, and ourselves.

As your baby grows, you'll need fewer supplies and you won't have to leave the house with a diaper bag that feels like the equivalent of a small shipping container. Your baby will go longer stretches of time between feedings and, yes, they will sleep. Your breasts won't feel engorged and ready to burst, and you'll be ready, willing, and eager to leave the house. You'll go out to dinner without your baby and maybe even leave town for a weekend. All of that will happen once you reach Oz.

And when it comes time to start planning that first birthday party, you'll notice that a lot of the baby struggles have been replaced with something new: toddler trials and tribulations. Yes, that little baby of yours will quickly grow into a curious and sometimes uncontrollable toddler, which will serve as your welcome to the next stage of parenthood. Prepare to wrestle your greasy little pig into a car seat. Get ready to carry your toddler surfboard-style as you flee from a public venue after an epic meltdown. As I said, the challenges don't go away; they just change as your child grows.

Becoming a mom has been the best thing I've ever done. That's not to say that it's easy, though. Parenting is like an endless game of whack-a-mole: You knock down one especially challenging phase and three more pop up. The game never ends.

You can't play the game if you're running on empty. You'll have nothing to give anyone, including your child. And, trust me, your baby will need a lot. But guess what? So do you!

Helpful Lists to
Save Your Sanity

I've never been big on making lists but when it came to giving birth and all things motherhood, I suddenly felt an overwhelming urge to be prepared for anything—and it became a newfound obsession. Since then, I've expanded and fine-tuned them, as a result of both my experiences and endless conversations with other new moms. The outcome here is a collection of exhaustive lists to make your dreams come true.

The Ultimate Hospital Packing List

S ure, you can easily google "hospital packing list" and you'll have endless options, but I've taken it a step further. Not only have I read and evaluated almost every list out there, but I've also spoken with hundreds of moms to help you prepare for just about anything. Yes, you need a large suitcase.

Documentation and Paperwork

- A photo ID and your health insurance card.

- Insurance papers and hospital paperwork you may have filled out in advance. For example, I had a scheduled C-section and was required to pay a certain percentage in advance, and also bring documentation from the hospital office verifying payment when I was admitted. (By the way, I forgot to do this, and my husband had to run down to the office to get a copy of the papers while I sat around and twiddled my thumbs, waiting to be admitted.)

- A few copies of your birth plan for your doctor and medical team. This way they'll know what you want and need since it's easy to forget in moments of pain and agony.

- Cord blood collection kit for your doctor, if you plan to bank it. Cord blood banking should be arranged around the third trimester. Once you have picked the company you will use and have signed up, they will send you the kit that you'll need to bring to the hospital.

- An advance medical directive, either in writing or shared with your partner or family. While it's unlikely, there is always the chance that things can go wrong. This directive will state your wishes about medical care should you become unable to make that decision yourself.

Clothing

- A robe. Hospital gowns are often open in the back. I was glad to have a robe to wear once I was able to stand up and walk so no one had to see my mesh underwear and diaper. I'd like to think everyone else appreciated that as well.

- **A nightgown/loungewear or personal hospital gown.** Some women don't like the hospital gowns and prefer their own comfortable clothing. Personally, I was more inclined to get the hospital's gown bloody than my own.

- **Large socks.** The hospital will likely provide you with those cozy socks with the plastic grips on the bottom, but you may want your own. I assumed I'd be given socks and wasn't or, rather, I didn't ask, and my feet were freezing before delivery.

- **Nursing or sleep bra.** Whether you plan to breastfeed or not, your milk will come in and your breasts will be big and sore. Be sure to pack a comfortable bra.

- **Extra underwear.** I loved the mesh granny panties from the hospital; in fact, I took extras home with me and was sad when I ran out. Not everyone loves them, and you won't know until you try. As a backup, bring extra underwear.

- **Slippers, flip-flops, or other comfortable (and stretchable) shoes.** Eventually, you'll want to walk around and those hospital floors are cold (and not exactly sterile). Again, just be sure they can accommodate any possible swelling. The same goes for any shoes you plan to wear home.

- **Going-home clothes.** Unless you want to leave in your hospital gown, anything relaxed and comfortable will work, such as a loose maternity dress. There is always a chance of an emergency C-section, so keep that in mind when packing.

- **Two sets of baby clothes.** The hospital will provide you with baby diapers, and generally a shirt, hat, and swaddle blankets. But you may have something special you'd like your child to wear home. The second set is just in case the first set gets too dirty (it probably will).

Toiletries

Essentials

- Toothbrush, dental floss, and toothpaste

- Shampoo, conditioner, and soap/body wash

- Nipple cream if you plan to breastfeed

- Lip balm

- Body lotion

- Hairbrush

- Hair ties/clips or headband

Optional

- Dry shampoo

- Face-cleaning wipes

- **Bath towels and washcloths.** The hospital will provide these, but some people prefer their own, sometimes due to detergent allergies.

- **Toilet paper/flushable wipes.** The toilet paper in the hospital is often single-ply and painful. Especially if you developed any hemorrhoids during pregnancy.

- **Postpartum care items:** Dermaplast spray, Tucks wipes, hemorrhoid cream, laxatives, and peri bottle.

- **Adult diapers.** What many moms refer to as their "diaper" is actually a pair of mesh underwear with an extra-large maxi pad. Many brands make what is called an "incontinence diaper," which is essentially a fancier version of what you will be given at the hospital.

Miscellaneous Items

- **Extra-long charging cord.** Hospitals aren't hotels. They're not designed for maximum comfort and ease, or optimal access to electrical outlets. You may find you need to charge your phone and the nearest outlet is across the room.

- **Snacks.** Yes, you will be fed in the hospital, but snacks are great for in between meals or when you wake up at 2 a.m. to feed your baby and realize that you're starving.

- **Bottled water.** The hospital will, of course, give you water, but you might have a La Croix flavor preference, which is perfectly reasonable.

- **Small cash bills and change.** Many vending machines now accept credit cards, but not all of them.

- **Large water cup or reusable bottle.** You'll need to be drinking a lot of water after you give birth. Not every hospital provides something big enough for a new mom's needs.

- **Nursing pillow.** I found this not only helpful for breastfeeding, but also because I was so sore from my C-section and it prevented my midsection from feeling the full effect of any sudden movements by serving as a barrier.

- **A pillow from home.** I was so tired I would have slept on the floor, but I know some people need their personal pillow to sleep.

- **Sheets and pillowcase.** I really didn't even notice the sheets, but some moms like to bring their own for a pop of color and comfort. You'll want to check with the hospital on size (twin, extra-long, etc.) and know that they may become stained with blood.

- **Book/tablet/laptop/handheld video game.** No, you won't feel much like reading after you give birth, but labor can be lengthy, and you might want to find a way to help pass the time.

- **Portable fan.** I wasn't especially hot after giving birth, but many women are. And it can be hard to regulate the temperature in a hospital room.

- **Eye mask.** People will be coming in and out of your room constantly, even at night. If you are sensitive to the light being turned on and off, you could benefit from an eye mask.

- **Earplugs/sound machine.** You may find yourself wanting to sleep during the day, but the noise around you prevents that. Both of these work well to muffle some of the noise, while still allowing you to hear your baby cry.

- **Night-light.** You may be able to avoid some, though probably not all, of the disturbance of fluorescent overhead lights by bringing a night-light.

- **A thank-you gift for your nurses.** As the daughter of a nurse and a friend of several nurses, I can tell you firsthand how hard they work for you. It's an especially personal relationship and you will be amazed at how comfortable they will make you feel as they tend to your uterus. I gave my nurses a box of candy on the day we were discharged, though after all they did to help, I felt like a new car would have been a more appropriate gift!

Questions to Ask About Your Health Before You Leave the Hospital

Take advantage of all the various experts working in the hospital while you can because it's highly unlikely that you'll be able to bribe any of them to come home with you to help. Take notes (or ask a family member or friend to do so), and ignore anyone who makes you feel like you're asking too much because these questions are about the MOM. Yes, so much about hospital discharge is about the baby, but it also is about you. Don't let anyone tell you differently.

- How do I care for my perineal or episiotomy stitches, or C-section incision?

- Will my stitches fall out? If so, when? And what if one pops out early?

- Has my breast milk come in yet? How will I be able to tell when it has?

- How will I know if I have a clogged milk duct or mastitis? And what should I do if I think I have either? Can I do anything to prevent these from happening?

- Can you provide me with tips for breastfeeding, including how to alleviate sore and chapped nipples?

- Do I have to be careful when lifting heavy items? Is there a weight restriction?

- Is it safe to use the stairs?

- How much bleeding is normal?

- How much pain is normal?

- What physical symptoms should be of concern?

- Do I need to continue taking my prenatal vitamins?

- Are there any over-the-counter medications I shouldn't take?

- What, if any, special nutritional needs do I need to be aware of? And what foods should I avoid?

- How much water should I drink each day?

- May I drink caffeinated beverages?

- May I drink alcohol?

- How active should I be at home the first week? And the second?

- May I drive my car?

- Who do I call if I have questions, or if I'm worried something is wrong?

- Are there extra mesh panties or pads I can take home?

The Essential Postpartum Bathroom Kit

L abor and delivery can be scary, but equally fear-inducing is a postpartum visit to the bathroom. To prepare, gather the following items that will provide the additional comfort when you need to use the toilet. You can put them in a bin or basket. The container doesn't need to be fancy because this won't live in your bathroom forever. I've made kits for friends who are expecting, using baskets from a dollar store large enough to hold all of these essential items.

- **Peri bottle.** This is a plastic bottle with an angled tip, which you use to squirt warm water on all your parts to clean yourself after using the bathroom, and it will be your new best friend. Because wiping will be terrifying.

- **Dermoplast.** This will come in handy for women who've had a vaginal birth. It's a pain-numbing spray that comes in an aerosol can. The main ingredient is benzocaine, and it will numb your screaming vag.

- **Industrial-strength maxi pads.** Find the absolute biggest and most absorbent pads available. That's usually an overnight-style, bonus if it has wings. The more coverage, the better.

- **Tucks cooling pads.** These wipes are marketed for hemorrhoids (which you also may be suffering from), but the soothing witch hazel makes them a perfect postpartum treat. You can lay these directly atop your massive maxi pad for cooling relief.

- **Extra underwear.** The blood is especially intense those first few days, so you'll be changing your underwear often.

- **Wet wipes.** Eventually, you will be able to wipe again, and you'll want to ease back into it with something softer than toilet paper.

- **Sanitizing wipes.** You may not make it to the toilet in time, and there might be blood. Don't bother getting a mop and toilet brush each time. Have something for a quick cleanup.

Everything—and I Mean EVERYTHING—to Discuss with Your Partner Before Your Baby Is Born

So many big and small details can slip through the cracks when your focus shifts to parenthood. You don't want that to happen with your partner because that's when pettiness sets in, tensions brew, and your relationship starts to unravel. So, do both of you a favor and have the talk when you are calm, clearheaded, and rested (aka, before the baby arrives).

Hospital

- Do you want visitors in the hospital? If so, who? Do you want to limit the length of visits? (Make a note to revisit this after your baby is born. You may feel differently then.)

- Will your partner spend the night in the hospital? Go home to nap?

- Who will stay in the hospital with you if not your partner?

- What if there is an emergency in the delivery room, or afterward? What is your medical directive for both mom and baby?

Coming Home

- How will you be bringing baby home? Car, taxi, etc.?

- How do you want to handle visitors at home? Should you limit the time they are there? Will you ask visitors to wash their hands first? Wear a mask? Do you want to allow anyone, or just close family and friends at first? (Make a note to revisit this after your baby is born. You may feel differently then.)

- What do you want to eat for the first week (at least)? Do you want to cook, order in food, get take-out fast food, use meal delivery kits, or have family/friends bring over food?

- How/when will you stock the pantry when you first come home? Who will make the grocery list and do the shopping? Will someone go to the grocery store? If so, who? Will you order groceries online? Who will place the order?

- Who will tackle miscellaneous household chores? If you have a C-section, you can count yourself out for a few weeks. What are your must-do chores around the house? Can any of them wait a week or so?

- Who will feed/walk/care for your pet(s)?

- How will you ensure that you both get enough sleep? Nap schedule? Take turns with nights?

Baby Needs

- Will you take turns with night wakings? If so, what will the schedule look like?

- Who will change the diapers?

- Who will pay for diapers? Will you buy in-store or online, and whose responsibility is that?

- Who will empty the diaper pail?

- If you are using bottles, who will wash them?

- Who will be responsible for buying the next size bottles as your baby grows?

- Who will wash, fold, and put away your baby's laundry?

- Who will give your baby their bath? Will you take turns, or do it together?

- Who will keep track of what size clothes your baby is wearing, and switch out clothes when your baby moves to the next size?

- Who will make pediatrician appointments? Who will take your baby to these appointments? Who will manage your baby's medical needs?

- Who will write and send out thank-you cards for the baby gifts you'll receive?

Mom Needs

- What do you expect from your partner while you're recovering?

- Do you want to breastfeed, bottle-feed, or do a combination of both? If breastfeeding, do you want to set a timeline for trying if you encounter challenges?

Are you both open to switching to formula if that is best for Mom?

- Do you plan to pump? If so, who will handle getting the breast pump through insurance or the hospital?

- If you breastfeed, will you also pump and use bottles? If so, will your partner help with feedings even at night? Will your partner help clean bottles and pump parts?

- What if you begin to experience baby blues or postpartum depression? Do you each understand what they are, and the difference between the two? Do you have a list of signs to be aware of?

Parenting

- If you are having a boy, what are your thoughts on circumcision?

- What does having an "active and engaged relationship" with your child look like to each of you? Both as a baby and throughout childhood.

- Do you want to raise your child in a certain religion?

- How do you want to celebrate birthdays and holidays?

- Which aspects from your own childhood do you want to incorporate into your role as a parent? Which do you want to avoid?

- What type of rules will you have for your child? What are your views on discipline?

- Are you interested in sleep training, or against it entirely?

- Do you want to set any boundaries with your families?

- How do you want to handle unsolicited advice? Ignore it? Share it with one another and evaluate?

- What are your expectations of grandparents and other family members?

- What are your plans for schooling? Public, private, religious?

- Do you want to share photos of your child on social media? If so, will your pages be public or private? Which platforms do you want to use?

- If you both work, who will stay home/take a day off to be home with your child when they are sick?

- If you both will be working, what are your plans for childcare?

- If one of you goes back to work and one of you stays home with your baby, how will that look? Will it shift the household responsibilities? How will the stay-at-home parent get breaks?

- Will you both hold the "mental load" that is required with a child? Who will keep track of various doctors' appointments and school forms?

- Will you make to-do lists together and carry them out? Or will one person make all the lists and the other follow their lead?

- Who will you call when you need help? A family member? Friend? Who do you *not* want to call?

- How long do you each want to try a system, solution, or product before you move on to something else if it isn't working?

Household Needs

- Who will clean the house moving forward? Will one of you watch the baby while the other cleans?

Set aside one day a week for housecleaning, or hire a housecleaning service?

- Who will be responsible for any pets after the baby is born?

- What do you plan to do for meals in the first few months with your new baby at home? Who will cook? Do you plan to eat dinners together as usual, or make quick meals?

- Do you have a family budget? Who will handle the finances?

Relationship

- What are you each willing to adjust from your pre-baby life to make more time for your child and family?

- How will you get time together alone and away from your baby?

- How will you each get alone time?

- What do you each really need for yourself? Gym time? Time at home while your partner takes the baby out?

- Will you each be willing to go to counseling if you feel that your relationship is suffering?

- Is your partner willing to go to therapy without you?

- How long will you wait as a couple before seeing a therapist?

- Will you make it a point to regularly check in with one another and see how the other is feeling?

- What is the plan for staying physically connected, such as handholding or cuddling, if you're not ready for sex?

- Are there affirmations that would reassure your partner that you still feel an attraction?

A Comprehensive List
of Childcare Considerations

Deciding on childcare can be an extensive, exhaustive, and emotional process, even more so if you don't know where to start. I polled experts in the field for suggestions that will help you begin your search and leave you more time to cuddle your baby (or sleep).

Budget

- What is your annual budget for childcare? What amount is at the top of your budget?

- If you plan to hire an in-home caregiver, does your budget allow for a competitive hourly rate and paid time off (sick leave, vacation time, paid holidays, etc.)?

- Does your budget allow for any unexpected costs that may arise throughout the year, such as fees, raises, or monetary investments?

- Does your budget allow for backup care to cover times when your primary caregiver is unavailable?

Your Child's Individual Needs

- Does your child have food allergies? Can they be accommodated? Where is the food prepared, and is there a chance of cross-contamination?

- Does your child need to be potty-trained?

- If your child is in diapers, how often do they change them? Do they specifically check each child or just follow a set schedule of diaper changes? If your child is being potty-trained at home, will they be able to help with that when your child is in their care?

- Does your child need to have medication administered to them during the day?

- Does your child have any other special needs or allergies, and can they be accommodated?

- What language do you speak at home? If you live in a multilingual home, do you have a language preference for your caregiver?

- Do you have any religious or cultural practices you want your caregiver to accommodate?

- Will your child be exposed to any animals, such as a caregiver's personal pet or class pets?

Safety

- What type of licenses and certifications does the facility and staff have, and are they current?

- Have background checks been run on all staff?

- Is every staff member CPR-certified?

- What is the policy on immunizations?

- Can the facility provide references that you can personally call and speak with?

- What is the emergency preparedness plan?

- What is the policy on visitors?

- How often is the facility cleaned and sanitized?

- What is your family's personal Covid protocol?

- What is the sick policy? Does your child have to stay home with a runny nose or fever?

- If you're hiring an individual caregiver, what is their protocol when your child is sick?

- Is there a specific nap area? What does it look like and where will your child sleep?

- What is your social media policy? Do you want your child excluded from any photos that may be used on the caregiver's website or social media?

Logistics

- What is the child-to-caregiver ratio?

- What hours do you need childcare? Do you need full- or part-time care?

- Do you need special or extended hours? If so, can that be accommodated? What is the additional cost?

- What is the late-pickup policy?

- Do you have any vacations planned? How much notice does the provider need? Do you still have to pay? Your contract should include a set number of days/weeks during the year that you will need care, and you should expect to pay for all scheduled days, even if you cancel care.

- Are there days when the provider won't be able to offer care, due to a vacation, holiday, or other needs?

- Do you need childcare on federal holidays?

- Are you responsible for your child's food and snacks? If not, what will be provided for them?

- Do you need to provide any supplies for your child?

- Do you have a preference for how phones and electronic communication are handled, such as whether the caregiver is only allowed to talk on the phone or text during breaks or naps? Remember: Your child also models what they see and it's reasonable to ask that they not be exposed to excessive technology use.

Curriculum

- What does a typical day look like?

- Is there an educational curriculum offered?

- What style of learning do you want for your child, such as nature- or play-based?

- Are there set goals for your child's learning?

- Do you want your child to have access to any specific subjects, such as language, arts, or music?

Practices and Protocols

- How is discipline approached?

- How are disruptive children handled? What is the bullying policy?

- Do you want the caregiver to offer or accept hugs from your child?

- How does the caregiver deal with children who are feeling scared? Sick? Emotional in general? Missing their parent(s)?

- How does the caregiver ease conflict between children, or between the child and the caregiver? Can they provide examples?

- How does the caregiver manage pressure? Can they provide examples?

Communication

- Is there a set schedule to check in on your child's progress? Can additional check-ins be scheduled?

- What form of communication is best for you, such as in-person, phone calls, or email? Does that work for the caregiver?

- Do you want to check in at any point during the day? Can the caregiver accommodate that?

- Does the caregiver write up accident reports if your child is injured, providing you with specific details? What constitutes an accident?

- Do you want a daily report of your child's behavior? Weekly?

- Would you prefer childcare that provides a live stream for parents?

Payment

- What is included in the contract?

- What is the payment schedule?

- What forms of payment are accepted, such as direct deposit, check, credit card?

- Will there be additional costs, separate from the base rate? If so, what? Is there a planned schedule?

- Will the caregiver agree to a paid trial period, after which both parties can decide if the relationship is a good fit and proceed with a contract?

Household Needs for At-Home Caregivers

- Have you informed your homeowner's insurance that someone will be working in your home?

- Do you need your caregiver to drive? If so, will you provide a car? Does your caregiver have a valid driver's license and proof of insurance? Can they supply you with a copy of their driving record?

- Do you want this person to cook for your child?

- Will you provide food and snacks for your caregiver or do you want them to bring in their own?

- What does the caregiver include in the scope of work? The industry standard is a "leave it as you found it" policy, meaning they will clean up after the child throughout the day, but nothing beyond that.

- Do you have household needs you expect this person to help with? Anything extra, such as dog walking, running your personal errands, and tasks not related directly to your child need to be compensated.

- Would you like your caregiver to take your child to any classes, such as music or a gym?

- Do you have specific wants for your child's schedule throughout the day? Such as getting outside for a walk, going to the park, or attending story time at the local library?

- Will you be restricting this person from having friends over to your home while they are working?

- How much advance notice would you like for non-emergency time off?

At-Home Hacks to Soothe Your Nethers

In addition to the many items on the market that can help you manage the physical pain and irritation caused by childbirth, there are two DIY treatments that many moms swear by. You can make these ahead of time during your final weeks of pregnancy, and that way you'll have icy treats at the ready when you return home.

Padsicles

A padsicle is a frozen maxi pad that can help with pain, soreness, and inflammation. They can be customized with ingredients known to soothe the skin, such as witch hazel or aloe vera. However, it's always a good idea to talk with your doctor before exposing that area of your body to any product. Also, if you've never used aloe vera gel or witch hazel topically, this probably isn't the right time to experiment. When in doubt, stick with water.

To make them you'll need:

    1 package of super-absorbent maxi pads

    1 roll of aluminum foil

Alcohol-free witch hazel or water

Freezer storage bags

100% aloe vera gel (optional)

Instructions:

1. Place each pad on a piece of aluminum foil large enough to wrap around the pad.

2. Pour the witch hazel or water over the pad. Be sure not to oversaturate the pad, otherwise it won't be able to absorb any blood or urine while you're wearing it.

3. At this point, you can also add a dollop of aloe vera gel to each pad if you'd like.

4. Once you have prepared all the pads, wrap each individually in foil so they won't stick together once frozen. Place them in a freezer storage bag in the freezer and let the magic happen.

How to use a padsicle:

Remove one padsicle from your freezer stash and let it thaw for a few minutes, because it will be literally freezing. Apply the pad adhesive to your underwear or adult diaper. If you added witch hazel and/or aloe vera gel, you will continue to benefit from the pad even after the chill wears off.

Condsicles

Yes, these are condom Popsicles. No, you won't need to insert them. These are for external use only. Condsicles are the perfect shape and size to sit upon, and they conform to the space between your legs—unlike ice packs, which tend to be awkwardly sized for that area.

To make them you'll need:

1 package nonlubricated condoms (use latex-free if you have an allergy)

Water

Aluminum foil

Freezer storage bags

Instructions:

1. Fill each condom with water, then tie them off as you would a water balloon.

2. Wrap each individually in aluminum foil so they won't stick together once frozen.

3. Place them in freezer storage bags and store in your freezer.

How to use a condsicle:

Like with any ice pack, your skin should not have direct contact with a condsicle, which could cause frostbite. Place a clean washcloth between your skin and the condsicle. Alternatively, cut a hole at the end of a panty liner and insert the condsicle between the layers. Apply the panty liner adhesive to your underwear or adult diaper. Condsicles will generally last around 20 minutes.

Resources and Further Reading

General Information for You and Your Baby's Health

BOOKS

Good Moms Have Scary Thoughts, by Karen Kleiman, MSW, and Molly McIntyre (Familius, 2019)

The Happiest Baby on the Block; Fully Revised and Updated Second Edition: The New Way to Calm Crying and Help Your Newborn Baby Sleep Longer, by Harvey Karp, MD (Bantam, 2015)

Self-Love Workbook for Women: Release Self-Doubt, Build Self-Compassion, and Embrace Who You Are, by Megan Logan, MSW, LCSW (Rockridge Press, 2020)

The Simplest Baby Book in the World: The Illustrated, Grab-and-Do Guide for a Healthy, Happy Baby, by Stephen Gross (The Simplest Company, 2021)

There Are Moms Way Worse Than You: Irrefutable Proof That You Are Indeed a Fantastic Parent, by Glenn Boozan (Workman Publishing Company, 2022)

ONLINE PUBLICATIONS

BabyCenter
www.babycenter.com
Provides pregnancy and parenting information from experts and also offers weekly emails tracking your baby's development, from conception to eight years old.

Scary Mommy
www.scarymommy.com
Content and articles that celebrate all aspects of a mother's journey.

Safe in the Seat
www.safeintheseat.com
Provides everything you need to know about car seats, from buying to installing, and offers online safety courses for parents.

La Leche League International
www.llli.org
Information, resources, and support for breastfeeding.

Kids Health Blog with Dr. Dina Kulik
drdina.ca
A mom and pediatrician, along with her team, offers informative articles on essentially any topic.

The Sterling Life
www.thesterlinglife.com
Comprehensive support for pregnancy and postpartum.

PODCASTS

Good Inside with Dr. Becky
www.goodinside.com/podcast
A clinical psychologist and mom of three, Dr. Becky Kennedy answers real parenting questions and provides actionable guidance.

What Fresh Hell: Laughing in the Face of Motherhood
www.whatfreshhellpodcast.com
With three episodes each week, this podcast features expert interviews and makes moms laugh. A lot.

The Mom Hour
themomhour.com/episodes
Hosted by two moms providing encouragement, community, and practical tips.

Websites, Hotlines, and Resources

HOSPITAL, LABOR, AND DELIVERY
Child and Baby First Aid/CPR AED★ by the American Red Cross
www.redcross.org
An online class to learn how to recognize and care for a variety of first aid, breathing, and cardiac emergencies. For in-person classes, ask your doctor or local hospital for recommendations.

American College of Obstetrics and Gynecologists

acog.org

Provides assistance for planning your labor and delivery, and covers everything you'll want to learn about childbirth.

POSTPARTUM PHYSICAL AND MENTAL HEALTH

Postpartum Support International

www.postpartum.net

Connects you with local resources, offers online support groups and information about postpartum mental health. You can also call the PSI helpline at 1-800-944-4773 for assistance in English or Spanish, or text "HELP" to 800-944-4773 for English or 971-203-7773 for Spanish.

The National Suicide Prevention Lifeline

www.988lifeline.org

Provides free and confidential mental health crisis services 24/7 for anyone in distress. Call 988 or 1-800-273-TALK (8255).

National Maternal Mental Health Hotline

www.mchb.hrsa.gov/national-maternal-mental-health-hotline

Provides free and confidential 24/7 support to women before, during, or after pregnancy, including phone or text access to counselors, local resources, and referrals. Call 1-833-9-HELP4MOMS (1-833-943-5746).

SLEEP AND SAFE SLEEP PRACTICES

American Academy of Pediatrics: Safe Sleep

www.aap.org/en/patient-care/safe-sleep

Evidence-based education and guidance for safe sleep practices.

The Wonder Weeks app

www.thewonderweeks.com/about-the-wonder-week-app/

Tracks a baby's developmental leaps and provides parents with ways to support them during these phases, especially when it affects sleep.

FOR ASSISTANCE WITH FORMULA, FOOD, AND OTHER ESSENTIALS

Women, Infants, and Children

www.fns.usda.gov/wic

Provides supplemental foods, health care referrals, and nutrition education for low-income women who are pregnant or post-partum, and for infants and children up to age five who are found to be at nutritional risk.

Supplemental Nutrition Assistance Program

www.fns.usda.gov/snap/state-directory

Provides nutritional benefits to eligible low-income individuals and families.

The National Diaper Bank Network

nationaldiaperbanknetwork.org

Call 2-1-1, a twenty-four-hour hotline that can help you identify local resources and learn about eligibility.

Cribs for Kids
cribsforkids.org

Provides free cribs for qualifying families and connects families with local agencies to apply for a free crib. They also offer online resources on safe sleep practices for parents.

Safe Kids Worldwide
www.safekids.org

A resource for free or low-cost car seats for eligible families.

Head Start Programs
www.acf.hhs.gov/ohs

Part of the US Department of Health and Human Services, available programs include childcare and free learning and development services for children from birth through age five.

Buy Nothing Project
buynothingproject.org

An international program hosted almost entirely on Facebook, where members can give, receive, share, and lend items among their neighbors, which may include food, clothes, toys, accessories, diapers, cribs, car seats, and bouncers.

CONNECT WITH OTHER MOMS

Peanut
www.peanut-app.io

An app for women to meet and connect with others who are at a similar stage in life.

Nextdoor
www.nextdoor.com

An app that connects you with your neighbors. You can search or post to find information about mom groups, local children/family events, or even to meet other moms. Also a useful resource for finding low- or no-cost. essentials, including clothes, toys, cribs, and strollers.

CHILDCARE

Find Child Care
www.childcare.gov

Directs you to your state's childcare search website.

Winnie
www.winnie.com

A marketplace to find local childcare providers. You can also view current licensing status, in-depth insights on providers, and enrollment information.

Care.com
www.care.com

Provides services and tools to help parents find, manage, and pay for care and make more informed hiring decisions about childcare.

References

Introduction

MacDorman M. F., E. Declercq. "Trends and state variations in out-of-hospital births in the United States, 2004-2017." *Birth* 46, no. 2 (June 2019): 279–288.

pubmed.ncbi.nlm.nih.gov/30537156/

Chapter 3

Centers for Disease Control and Prevention. Breastfeeding report card: United States, 2022. U.S. Department of Health & Human Services.

www.cdc.gov/breastfeeding/pdf/2022-Breastfeeding-Report-Card-H.pdf

Chapter 5

Karney, B. R., N. E. Frye. "'But we've been getting better lately': Comparing prospective and retrospective views of relationship development." *Journal of Personality and Social Psychology*, 82, no. 2 (2002): 222–238.

doi.org/10.1037/0022-3514.82.2.222

References

Chapter 6

Burnham, M. M., B. L. Goodlin-Jones, E. E. Gaylor, T. F. Anders. "Nighttime sleep-wake patterns and self-soothing from birth to one year of age: a longitudinal intervention study," *Journal of Child Psychology and Psychiatry*, 43 (July 2002): 713-725. doi.org/10.1111/1469-7610.00076

Rivkees, S. A., M. Mirmiran, R. L. Ariagno. "Circadian Rhythms in Infants," *NeoReviews*, no. 11 (November 2003): e298-e304. doi.org/10.1542/neo.4-11-e298

Gold, J. "Sleeping like a baby is a $325 million industry," *Marketplace*, American Public Media, January 16, 2017. www.marketplace.org/2017/01/16/sleeping-baby-325-million-industry/

Chapter 8

Cleveland Clinic. "Lochia (Postpartum Bleeding): How Long, Stages, Smell & Color," *Cleveland Clinic Journal of Medicine*, Cleveland Clinic, March 11, 2022. my.clevelandclinic.org/health/symptoms/22485-lochia

Chapter 9

Bauman, B. L., J. Y. Ko, S. Cox, et al. "Postpartum Depressive Symptoms and Provider Discussions About Perinatal Depression." United States: 2018. Morbidity and Mortality Weekly Report 69, no. 19 (2002): 575-581. dx.doi.org/10.15585/mmwr.mm6919a2

References

Ko, J. Y., K. M. Rockhill, V. T. Tong, B. Morrow, S. L. Farr. "Trends in Postpartum Depressive Symptoms—27 States, 2004, 2008, and 2012." Morbidity and Mortality Weekly Report 66, no. 6 (2017): 153–158.
dx.doi.org/10.15585/mmwr.mm6606a1External

Byatt, N., et al. "Summary of Perinatal Mental Health Conditions." American College of Obstetrics and Gynecology (February 2022). https://www.acog.org/-/media/project/acog/acogorg/files/forms/perinatal-mental-health-toolkit/summary-of-perinatal-mental-health-conditions.pdf?la=en&hash=3FD8EEB5AD79D-9A49CD2600954A4EE8B

Chapter 12
Child Care Aware of America, "Demanding Change: Repairing our Child Care System" (Washington: 2022).
info.childcareaware.org/hubfs/FINAL-Demanding%20Change%20Report-020322.pdf

Acknowledgments

Jessica Firger, you are everything this book—and I—needed. To simply refer to you as my editor doesn't feel like enough. You've been my champion and I am honored to have worked with you.

Everyone at Union Square & Co. who added their personal magic, including Lindsay Herman, Rich Hazelton, and Melissa Farris. Thank you to Sara Wood, who designed the cover.

Joelle Delbourgo, my agent who understood my vision and fought like hell to not only get it published, but to make sure it was in the right hands.

The incomparable Jennie Nash, the queen of book coaches and North Star of my writing career. And to your team, the wonderful Lianne Scott and Vanessa Soto.

Michelle Dempsey-Multack, my dream became a reality because of your help and belief in me.

The brilliant experts who generously shared their time and knowledge with me: Marquis Anne, Dr. Alice Boyes, Leah Castro, Jessica Choi, Kerrin Edmonds, Dr. Morgan Francis,

Acknowledgments

Matthew Johnson, Dr. Dina Kulik, Dr. Christine Sterling, and Leslie Wasserman.

The women who bravely told me their personal stories for this book. I thank you for entrusting me with them.

All the moms who are in the trenches with me on Instagram and have supported me through the years. And the women who have become family: the snack-sized queens and the spill text squad.

Dina Freeman, Betsy Shaw, and Joyce Slaton Lollar of BabyCenter, who took a chance and hired a pregnant former publicist who had a story to tell and no idea how to do it.

Sam Angoletta, Joelle Wisler, and Karen Johnson of Scary Mommy, you saw something in me that I couldn't see myself and taught me to honor my voice.

Lin Manuel-Miranda, we'll likely never meet, but the songs of *Hamilton* sparked my passion to advocate for moms and inspired this book.

Judy Blume, you made me want to be an author. And showed me that I could do it.

My Walnut Acres friends who always let me know I had support and help. Elizabeth, there will never be enough song lyrics to express what you mean to me. Jamie, you literally kept me alive. You validate my thoughts and feelings and are my safe space. Kayla (my person), Brook and Soma, my first mom friends. Glenda, you are always with me and in this book. Marie,

Acknowledgments

my friend and talented researcher. Mimi, I could never have done this without your help, support, and endless encouragement. Best SW ever. Nicole, you make everything better. You cheer louder, listen harder, and care more than anyone. I'm so lucky. And grateful.

Mike and Susan "Strawberry" and Jason, the most supportive cousin-siblings. Grandma, I love you more. Jen, the best sister, protector, supporter, aunt, and one of Archie's favorite humans.

Mom and Dad. You've always believed in me and provided endless support and guidance at every turn. The best Ganma & Pop Pop that Archie could ask for. There is absolutely no way this could have happened without you both.

Mike. When I decided that I wanted to write this book you immediately said, "Do it!" No questions or hesitation, only complete support. Always. You are the best thing.

Archer Raymond. I know you wish this book was about toilet humor, but I hope that one day you'll be proud. Becoming your mom started my life anew, it taught me who I truly am and what I was meant to do. Thank you for choosing me from the "mommy store." I love you more than the whole universe and all of Joseph Eichler's inventions combined.

About the Author

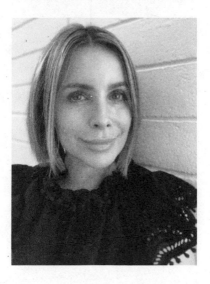

Becky Vieira is the voice behind the Instagram mom account @WittyOtter, where she is leading the shift in the way women speak about motherhood. For more than six years she has been a go-to writer in the parenting space for popular outlets including BabyCenter and Scary Mommy. Before becoming a writer, Vieira spent more than fifteen years as a publicist for some of the biggest public relations agencies representing major consumer brands, including Mattel's Barbie, Disney Consumer Products, and the charitable program Stand Up to Cancer. She lives in the San Francisco Bay Area with her husband, son, three cats, one dog, and a partridge in a pear tree.